Detection of SARS-CoV-2 Antibodies in Diagnosis and Treatment of COVID-19

Editors

DAIMON P. SIMMONS
PETER H. SCHUR

CLINICS IN LABORATORY MEDICINE

www.labmed.theclinics.com

Editor-In-Chief
MILENKO JOVAN TANASIJEVIC

March 2022 • Volume 42 • Number 1

ELSEVIER

1600 John F. Kennedy Boulevard ● Suite 1800 ● Philadelphia, Pennsylvania, 19103-2899

http://www.theclinics.com

CLINICS IN LABORATORY MEDICINE Volume 42, Number 1
March 2022 ISSN 0272-2712, ISBN-13: 978-0-323-83586-2

Editor: Katerina Heidhausen
Developmental Editor: Ann Gielou M. Posedio

Reprints. For copies of 100 or more, of articles in this publication, please contact the Commercial Reprints Department, Elsevier Inc., 360 Park Avenue South, New York, New York 10010-1710. Tel. 212-633-3874, Fax: 212-633-3820, E-mail: reprints@elsevier.com.

Clinics in Laboratory Medicine (ISSN 0272-2712) is published quarterly by Elsevier Inc., 360 Park Avenue South, New York, NY 10010-1710. Months of issue are March, June, September, and December. Business and Editorial offices: 1600 John F. Kennedy Blvd., Suite 1800, Philadelphia, PA 19103-2899. Periodicals postage paid at NewYork, NY and additional mailing offices. Subscription prices are $283.00 per year (US individuals), $753.00 per year (US institutions), $100.00 per year (US students), $363.00 per year (Canadian individuals), $776.00 per year (Canadian institutions), $100.00 per year (Canadian students), $404.00 per year (international individuals), $776.00 per year (international institutions), $185.00 (international students). Foreign air speed delivery is included in all Clinics subscription prices. All prices are subject to change without notice. POSTMASTER: Send address changes to *Clinics in Laboratory Medicine*, Elsevier Health Sciences Division, Subscription Customer Service, 3251 Riverport Lane, Maryland Heights, MO 63043. **Customer Service: 1-800-654-2452 (US). From outside of the US and Canada, call 1-314-447-8871. Fax: 1-314-447-8029. E-mail: journalscustomerservice-usa@elsevier.com (for print support) or journalsonlinesupport-usa@elsevier.com (for online support).**

Clinics in Laboratory Medicine is covered in *EMBASE/Exerpta Medica, MEDLINE/PubMed (Index Medicus), Cinahl, Current Contents/Clinical Medicine, BIOSIS and ISI/BIOMED.*

Contributors

EDITOR-IN-CHIEF

MILENKO JOVAN TANASIJEVIC, MD, MBA
Vice Chair for Clinical Pathology and Quality, Department of Pathology, Director of Clinical Laboratories, Brigham and Women's Hospital, Dana-Farber Cancer Institute, Associate Professor of Pathology, Harvard Medical School, Boston, Massachusetts, USA

EDITORS

DAIMON P. SIMMONS, MD, PhD
Department of Pathology, Brigham and Women's Hospital, Boston, Massachusetts, USA

PETER H. SCHUR, MD, MACR, MACP, MAAAS
Professor of Medicine, Harvard Medical School, Division of Rheumatology, Brigham and Women's Hospital, Boston, Massachusetts, USA

AUTHORS

LINDSEY R. BADEN, MD
Division of Infectious Diseases, Brigham and Women's Hospital, Harvard Medical School, Boston, Massachusetts, USA

CHI-AN CHENG, PhD
Department of Pathology, Brigham and Women's Hospital, Wyss Institute for Biologically Inspired Engineering, Harvard University, Harvard Medical School, Boston, Massachusetts, USA

MICHAËL DESJARDINS, MD
Division of Infectious Diseases, Brigham and Women's Hospital, Harvard Medical School, Boston, Massachusetts, USA; Division of Infectious Diseases, Centre Hospitalier de l'Université de Montréal, Montreal, Quebec, Canada

TAL GILBOA, PhD
Department of Pathology, Brigham and Women's Hospital, Wyss Institute for Biologically Inspired Engineering, Harvard University, Harvard Medical School, Boston, Massachusetts, USA

JESSE GITAKA, MB ChB, PhD
Directorate of Research and Innovation, Mount Kenya University, Thika, Kenya

SIDDHARTH KHARE, PhD
Micelio Labs, Bengaluru, India

ROEY LAZAROVITS, BS
Department of Pathology, Brigham and Women's Hospital, Wyss Institute for Biologically Inspired Engineering, Harvard University, Boston, Massachusetts, USA

VINAY S. MAHAJAN, MBBS, PhD
Ragon Institute of MGH, MIT and Harvard, Cambridge, Massachusetts, USA; Department of Pathology, Brigham and Women's Hospital, Boston, Massachusetts, USA

SAMUEL MUNGAI, MS
Directorate of Research and Innovation, Mount Kenya University, Thika, Kenya

LUCY OCHOLA, PhD
Department of Tropical and Infectious Diseases, Institute of Primate Research, National Museums of Kenya, Nairobi, Kenya

ALANA F. OGATA, PhD
Department of Pathology, Brigham and Women's Hospital, Wyss Institute for Biologically Inspired Engineering, Harvard University, Harvard Medical School, Boston, Massachusetts, USA

PAUL OGONGO, PhD
Department of Tropical and Infectious Diseases, Institute of Primate Research, National Museums of Kenya, Nairobi, Kenya; Division of Experimental Medicine, Department of Medicine, University of California, San Francisco, San Francisco, California, USA

RASHMI PATEL, MBBS, MS
Micelio Labs, Bengaluru, India

SHIV PILLAI, MBBS, PhD
Ragon Institute of MGH, MIT and Harvard, Professor of Medicine and Health Sciences and Technology, Harvard Medical School, Cambridge, Massachusetts, USA

AMY C. SHERMAN, MD
Division of Infectious Diseases, Brigham and Women's Hospital, Harvard Medical School, Boston, Massachusetts, USA

PATRICIA R. SLEV, PhD, D(ABCC)
Section Chief, Immunology Division, ARUP Laboratories, Associate Professor, Department of Pathology, University of Utah School of Medicine, Salt Lake City, Utah, USA

SARA SULIMAN, MPH, PhD
Division of Rheumatology, Inflammation and Immunity, Brigham and Women's Hospital, Boston, Massachusetts, USA; Division of Experimental Medicine, Department of Medicine, University of California, San Francisco, San Francisco, California, USA

ELITZA S. THEEL, PhD, D(ABMM)
Professor, Laboratory Medicine and Pathology, Director, Infectious Diseases Serology Laboratory, Co-Director, Vector-Borne Diseases Service Line, Division of Clinical Microbiology, Department of Laboratory Medicine and Pathology, Mayo Clinic, Rochester, Minnesota, USA

AUGUSTA UWAMANZU-NNA, BS
Department of Pathology, Brigham and Women's Hospital, Boston, Massachusetts, USA

DAVID R. WALT, PhD
Department of Pathology, Brigham and Women's Hospital, Wyss Institute for Biologically Inspired Engineering, Harvard University, Harvard Medical School, Boston, Massachusetts, USA

DUANE R. WESEMANN, MD, PhD
Department of Medicine, Divisions of Allergy and Immunology, and Genetics, Brigham and Women's Hospital, Harvard Medical School, Boston, Massachusetts, USA

ADAM ZUIANI, PhD
Department of Medicine, Divisions of Allergy and Immunology, and Genetics, Brigham and Women's Hospital, Harvard Medical School, Boston, Massachusetts, USA

Contents

In 2019, an emerging coronavirus, SARS-COV-2, was first identified. In the months since, SARS-CoV-2 has become a global pandemic of unimaginable scale. In 2021, SARS-CoV-2 continues to be a huge public health burden and a dominating issue in health care. In addition, SARS-CoV-2 has placed a spotlight on laboratory medicine and its key role in infectious disease management. The SARS-CoV-2 antibody testing landscape is vast and consists of dozens of antibody tests that have received EUA. The laboratory is faced with choosing the right test, staying current with the rapidly evolving recommendations, and updating test information for clients and clinicians. This review addresses what we know about the humoral response in SARS-CoV-2 infection and how this knowledge translates into appropriate serology test choice, utility, and interpretation.

This review provides a broad summary of the performance characteristics of high-throughput severe acute respiratory syndrome coronavirus 2 (SARS-CoV-2) serologic assays with Food and Drug Administration Emergency Use Authorization, which are commonly found in central clinical laboratories. In addition, this review discusses the current roles of serologic testing for SARS-CoV-2 and provides a perspective for the future.

The coronavirus disease of 2019 (COVID-19) pandemic, caused by infection with the severe acute respiratory syndrome coronavirus-2 (SARS-CoV-2), has undoubtedly resulted in significant morbidities, mortalities, and economic disruptions across the globe. Affordable and scalable tools to monitor the transmission dynamics of the SARS-CoV-2 virus and the longevity of induced antibodies will be paramount to monitor and control the pandemic as multiple waves continue to rage in many countries. Serologic assays detect humoral responses to the virus, to determine seroprevalence in target populations, or induction of antibodies at the individual level following either natural infection or vaccination. With multiple vaccines rolling out globally, serologic assays to detect anti-SARS-CoV-2 antibodies will be important tools to monitor the development of herd immunity. To address this need, serologic lateral flow assays (LFAs), which can be easily implemented for both population surveillance and home use, will be vital to monitor the evolution of the pandemic and inform containment measures. Such assays are particularly important for monitoring the transmission dynamics and durability of immunity generated by natural infections and vaccination, particularly in resource-limited settings. In this review, we discuss considerations for evaluating the accuracy of these LFAs, their suitability for different use cases, and implementation opportunities.

The COVID-19 pandemic has resulted in the development, validation, and rapid adoption of multiple novel diagnostic approaches. Hundreds of SARS-CoV-2 serologic assays have been developed and deployed to contain the spread of the virus, and to supply timely and important health information. Most of these serologic assays were based on a conventional enzyme-linked immunosorbent assay or the lateral flow assay format. The immunoassays that were developed were based on alternative technologies and are highlighted in this article with a brief discussion of the assay principle and the pros and cons for each assay. Measurement of neutralizing antibodies is also discussed.

This review describes the underlying basis for the sup-optimal humoral immune response in coronavirus disease (COVID)-19 including the absence of evidence for affinity maturation in the vast majority of patients and the absence of germinal centers even in severe disease. Suboptimal humoral and cellular immunity may provide the optimal conditions for the generation and selection of viral variants.

Severe acute respiratory syndrome coronavirus 2 (COVID)-19 has emerged as the greatest global health threat in generations. An unprecedented mobilization of researchers has generated a wealth of data on humoral responses to SARS-CoV-2 within a year of the pandemic's beginning. The rapidly developed understanding of acute-phase antibody induction and medium-term antibody durability in COVID-19 is important at an individual level to inform patient care and a population level to help predict transmission dynamics. In this brief review, we will describe the development and maintenance of antibody responses to immunization and infections generally and the specific antibody dynamics observed for COVID-19. These crucial features of the humoral response have implications for the use of antibody therapeutics against the virus and can inform the likelihood of reinfection of individuals by the virus.

Severe Acute Respiratory Syndrome Coronavirus 2 Antigens as Targets of Antibody Responses

Alana F. Ogata, Roey Lazarovits, Augusta Uwamanzu-Nna, Tal Gilboa, Chi-An Cheng, and David R. Walt

Humoral immunity to severe acute respiratory syndrome coronavirus 2 (SARS-CoV-2) during acute infection and convalescence has been widely studied since March 2020. In this review, the authors summarize literature on humoral responses to SARS-CoV-2 antigens with a focus on spike, nucleocapsid, and the receptor-binding domain as targets of antibody responses. They highlight serologic studies during acute SARS-CoV-2 infection and discuss the clinical relevance of antibody levels in COVID-19 progression. Antibody responses in pediatric COVID-19 patients are also reviewed. Finally, the authors discuss antibody responses during convalescence and their role in protection from SARS-CoV-2 reinfection.

Vaccine-Induced Severe Acute Respiratory Syndrome Coronavirus 2 Antibody Response and the Path to Accelerating Development (Determining a Correlate of Protection)

Amy C. Sherman, Michaël Desjardins, and Lindsey R. Baden

As new public health challenges relating to COVID-19 emerge, such as variant strains, waning vaccine efficacy over time, and decreased vaccine efficacy for special populations (immunocompromised hosts), it is important to determine a correlate of protection (CoP) to allow accurate bridging studies for special populations and against variants of concern. Large-scale phase 3 clinical trials are inefficient to rapidly assess novel vaccine candidates for variant strains or special populations, because these trials are slow and costly. Defining a practical CoP will aid in efficiently conducting future assessments to further describe protection for individuals and on a population level for surveillance.

CLINICS IN LABORATORY MEDICINE

SERIES OF RELATED INTEREST

Surgical Pathology Clinics
Available at: https://www.surgpath.theclinics.com/

THE CLINICS ARE NOW AVAILABLE ONLINE!
Access your subscription at:
www.theclinics.com

Preface

Perspectives on Antibodies Against Severe Acute Respiratory Syndrome Coronavirus 2 and Its Implications for Diagnostics, Biology, and Clinical Management

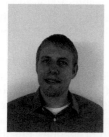 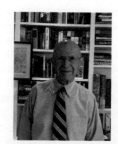

Daimon P. Simmons, MD, PhD   Peter H. Schur, MD, MACR, MACP, MAAAS

Editors

When the pandemic coronavirus disease 2019 (COVID-19) swept around the world in early 2020, diagnostic testing moved into the spotlight. Although molecular diagnostic tests have been a mainstay in identification of patients infected with the severe acute respiratory syndrome coronavirus 2 (SARS-CoV-2) virus, detection of viral nucleic acids may be limited to the initial phase of infection. Detection of anti-SARS-CoV-2 antibodies complements molecular testing as a method of detecting previously infected individuals. A large number of assays were rapidly released due to the urgent need for diagnostics in this pandemic, highlighting the need for rigorous quality control and assay evaluation. With more recent availability of vaccines, the diagnostic role of anti-SARS-CoV-2 antibody detection has shifted to distinguish natural infection from effective response to a vaccine. In this issue of *Clinics in Laboratory Medicine*, a breadth of reviews describe the role of antibodies in this pandemic but also provide unique perspectives about different aspects of serologic testing for SARS-CoV-2.

The reviews in this issue describe the timing and durability of antibody responses, which are critical factors in the interpretation of these serology results. The distinction between detection of binding antibodies and neutralizing antibodies that may confer clinical immunity is another important recurring theme. There are also important

Clin Lab Med 42 (2022) xi–xiii
https://doi.org/10.1016/j.cll.2021.12.001
0272-2712/22/© 2021 Published by Elsevier Inc.

perspectives that are shared between multiple reviews, including information and guidelines on the evaluation of different assays. Some articles detail the immunologic responses involved in immune responses to SARS-CoV-2, along with some that comment on implications of new SARS-CoV-2 variants. Finally, there are perspectives about the importance of antibodies in clinical management and vaccination.

There are many unique perspectives included among these reviews. In "Severe Acute Respiratory Syndrome Coronavirus 2 Serology Testing: A Laboratory Primer," Patricia Slev provides a general primer on the topic, including recommendations for assay evaluation. Elitza Theel describes differences in technical performance of different assays in "Performance Characteristics of High-Throughput Serologic Assays for Severe Acute Respiratory Syndrome Coronavirus 2 with Food and Drug Administration Emergency Use Authorization: A Review," mentioning the particular importance of high specificity in diagnostic testing. The article "Performance Evaluation of Lateral Flow Assays for Coronavirus Disease 2019 Serology" by Lucy Ochola and colleagues provides a perspective on cost-effective approaches, particularly lateral flow assays, to define seroprevalence globally. Rashmi Patel and colleagues expand on technical details of different antibody detection methods in their article, "Alternative Methods to Detect Severe Acute Respiratory Syndrome Coronavirus 2 antibodies." Shiv Pillai focuses on the biology of germinal center responses and the overly exuberant immune responses that impair B-cell responses in "Suboptimal Humoral Immunity in Severe Acute Respiratory Syndrome Coronavirus 2 Infection and Viral Variant Generation." In their article "Antibody Dynamics and Durability in Coronavirus Disease 2019," Adam Zuiani and Duane Wesemann describe the immunologic details of B-cell activation and development of effective antibodies related to COVID-19. Alana Ogata and colleagues describe clinical implications of anti-SARS-CoV-2 antibodies in the article "Coronavirus Antigens as Targets of Antibody Responses," including discussion of antibodies in diagnosis of pediatric inflammatory syndromes. The issue concludes with an article by Amy Sherman and colleagues, "Vaccine-induced Severe Acute Respiratory Syndrome Coronavirus 2 Antibody Response and the Path to Accelerating Development (Determining a Correlate of Protection)," with a focus on the interpretation of these antibodies in context of vaccines.

This issue of *Clinics in Laboratory Medicine* brings together important perspectives on antibodies against SARS-CoV-2, including immunology, infectious disease, clinical diagnostics, and clinical management. Anti-SARS-CoV-2 antibodies can reflect past infection of an individual with this virus, but they also help identify effective immune responses, either to viral infection or to vaccination. The shared perspectives and unique information provided in these review articles help to illuminate persistent questions and evolving knowledge about diagnostic testing in the COVID-19 pandemic.

Daimon P. Simmons, MD, PhD
Department of Pathology
Brigham and Women's Hospital
75 Francis Street
Boston, MA 02115, USA

Peter H. Schur, MD, MACR, MACP, MAAAS
Division of Rheumatology
Brigham and Women's Hospital
75 Francis Street
Boston, MA 02115, USA

E-mail addresses:
dsimmons4@bwh.harvard.edu (D.P. Simmons)
pschur@bwh.harvard.edu (P.H. Schur)

Severe Acute Respiratory Syndrome Coronavirus 2 Serology Testing – A Laboratory Primer

Patricia R. Slev, PhD, D(ABCC)[a,b,*]

KEYWORDS

- SARS-CoV-2 serology • COVID-19 • Antibody laboratory testing

KEY POINTS

- There are dozens of EUA serology assays,for SARS-CoV-2 that differ in methodology, antibody class detected, antigenic target, and performance characteristics. Although there are recommendations against using IgM as a standalone and IgA, there are no other specific recommendations with regard to antigenic target or antibody class.
- The vast majority of antibody assays are qualitative and detect binding antibodies which include neutralizing antibodies. There is one EUA serology assay that specifically detects neutralizing antibodies. Multiple studies have demonstrated a positive correlation between binding and neutralizing antibody assays.
- Antibody testing should not be used for diagnosing SARS-CoV-2 infection and utility is currently limited to seroprevalence studies, as an aid in supporting a multisystem inflammatory syndrome in children (MIS-C) diagnosis, or diagnosis in adults presenting late in the disease course, and identifying eligible donors for COVID-19 convalescent plasma (CCP).
- As of May 2021, there are no recommendations from any of the professional societies (IDSA, CDC, AACC) for antibody testing to qualify for vaccine administration postnatural infection or for assessing adequate immune response due to vaccination.

INTRODUCTION

In 2019, a new coronavirus virus, SARS-CoV-2, emerged that would lead to a worldwide pandemic and highlight the importance of laboratory medicine in infectious disease management.[1] In 2021, SARS-CoV-2 remains a priority for laboratory testing. Although diagnostic testing to determine who was infected with the virus was at the forefront of the pandemic, as serology testing became available, public interest in

[a] Immunology Division, ARUP Laboratories, 500 Chipeta Way, Salt Lake City, UT 80108, USA;
[b] Department of Pathology, University of Utah School of Medicine, Salt Lake City, UT, USA
* ARUP Laboratories, 500 Chipeta Way, Salt Lake City, UT 80108, USA
E-mail address: Patricia.slev@aruplab.com

Clin Lab Med 42 (2022) 1–13
https://doi.org/10.1016/j.cll.2021.10.003
0272-2712/22/© 2021 Elsevier Inc. All rights reserved.

labmed.theclinics.com

testing quickly rose and demanded that laboratories offer serology testing, even though antibody testing utility was limited. In the early days of the pandemic, March and April 2020, serology testing was not recommended for clinical purposes and was deemed of limited clinical value.[2,3] Therefore, the FDA did not see a need for strict regulations for antibody testing. This led to a proliferation of SARS-CoV-2 antibody tests, dominated early on by lateral flow assays (LFA) imported from various parts of the world. At the time, the FDA only required that the manufacturer notify the FDA of their intent to bring an antibody assay to market without any data requirements to support the performance characteristics of the assay. The consequence was a rapid and unprecedented proliferation of unvalidated, expensive assays quickly made available to anyone who wanted access. In addition, many were confused about rapid tests and incorrectly assumed that because of the ease of use that these rapid tests could be used in any setting, such as physicians' offices, without laboratory oversight or validation. The combination of public curiosity as to whether they had been infected with the virus and the lack of validated antibody tests used indiscriminately in any setting was accompanied by a considerable amount of bad press because many of the assays were inaccurate. This situation quickly escalated and highlighted the need for quality serology tests, FDA oversight, and the importance of the laboratory in validating serology assays. In early May 2020, the FDA issued new guidance for Emergency Use Authorization (EUA) claims for serology assays, that stated that, although manufacturers could notify the FDA of their intent to bring a serology assay to market as a first step to obtaining EUA, the manufacturer also had to provide supporting data to the FDA within 10 days of the notification. In addition, the FDA instituted an umbrella protocol that allowed for serology assays to be independently evaluated through NIH by agencies such as the National Cancer Institute (NCI), CDC, and Biomedical Advanced Research and Development Authority (BARDA). The FDA has also published templates for test manufacturers with recommendations for the number of samples that should be evaluated to determine performance characteristics and threshold requirements for performance characteristics (please refer to the section on serology assay evaluation).

The pandemic and serology testing have rapidly evolved and today we have a plethora of EUA serology assays available, and the list is still growing every day. There have been 21 new serology assays approved just since January 1, 2021. The good news is that many advances have been made and there are many high-quality assays but there is now increased confusion about test choice, test utility, and test result interpretation. The SARS-CoV-2 EUA serology testing landscape has been recently reviewed by Ravi and colleagues.[4] Confusion is driven not just by a large number of assay options but also by the rapidly evolving science about antibody kinetics, antibody durability, and protective immunity in the context of SARS-CoV-2 infection and now, vaccination.

SEVERE ACUTE RESPIRATORY SYNDROME CORONAVIRUS 2 HUMORAL RESPONSE
Not All Antibodies Are Created Equal

One concept that is not typically highlighted for other infectious diseases as far as the choice of serologic assay that has become critical to our understanding of SARS-CoV-2 infection is the different categories of antibodies and their role in the adaptive immune response. All antibodies bind to an antigen and serve a role in clearing infection. However, binding antibodies consist of both nonneutralizing and neutralizing antibodies (Nabs). Non-Nabs typically develop before Nabs and may function in viral clearance but do not extinguish infective virus. In contrast, there is a category of binding antibodies that are referred to as Nabs that can be of various antibody classes and have the unique ability to prevent cellular infection, potentially limiting initial infection and disease severity, as well as possibly preventing reinfection. For example, in the case of SARS-CoV-2 infection, Nabs develop that bind to the receptor-binding domain (RBD) region of the virus, thereby interfering with the virus's ability to interact with the angiotensin-converting enzyme 2 (ACE2) cellular receptor on the cell surface and thereby preventing cellular infection.[5–10] The typical laboratory antibody assays measure binding antibodies, without distinguishing between neutralizing and non-Nabs. Although Nab assays provide a functional indication of the immune system and may correlate with protective immunity, it is not established what concentration of Nabs confers protective immunity due to natural infection or vaccination.

Due to the role of Nabs, many studies have investigated a correlation between commercial serology assays that measure binding antibodies and neutralization assay results. There is a general qualitative agreement and a positive correlation between binding and Nab assays. Studies also show that not surprisingly, there is a higher degree of correlation between Nab assays and binding antibody assays that use the spike protein as a target.[11–13] Nab concentrations provide important information about levels of functional antibody and have been used in vaccine development; however, there are currently no recommendations for the clinical use of neutralization assays to specifically assess vaccine response, determine infection risk or predict disease severity.[14–16]

Antibody Kinetics and Durability

Although we continue to learn about the fine details of the humoral response against SARS-CoV-2 as the pandemic unfolds, we do have a basic understanding of the antibody response in SARS-CoV-2 infection. The majority of studies indicate that infected individuals mount a SARS-CoV-2 specific antibody response in the acute stage of the disease and over 90% of infected individuals have detectable antibodies 3-weeks postsymptom onset. For IgM, the time to seroconversion ranges from 4 to 14 days.[17] Mean time to seroconversion for IgG is 12 to 15 days, and generally detectable 7 to 14-days postsymptom onset. For IgA, most studies suggest seroconversion within 4-days postsymptom onset. IgM and IgG develop almost simultaneously without a significant delay between detectable IgM and IgG.[18] The majority of studies demonstrate that IgM peaks 2 to 5-weeks postsymptom onset, and rapidly declines thereafter. IgA is less well studied but also seems to decline within a few weeks postinfection.

Early studies suggested that IgG antibody responses waned rapidly during the convalescent stage[18] and that IgG may not be durable, particularly in individuals who experienced mild forms of COVID-19.[19] More recent studies suggest that the IgG antibody response postnatural infection is detectable during the convalescent stage, and although IgG levels decline over time and may vary with disease severity, an IgG response can remain detectable up to several months, with at least one study reporting detection of RBD-spike IgG seropositivity in 88% of individuals at 8-months postinfection.[17,20–22] Studies also indicate that 4% to 10% of infected individuals may have undetectable or a delayed antibody response following SARS-CoV-2 infection.[22]

Nab titers have been shown to correlate with disease severity, and individuals with a more severe form of disease had higher titers of Nabs.[17,23–25] Most studies demonstrated that Nabs are detectable between 7 and 15-days postsymptom onset and most individuals were positive by 21-days postdisease onset.[26] Although asymptomatic individuals had lower antibody titers, Nab titers varied considerably between individuals.[24] Furthermore, although disease severity affected the magnitude of the Nab response, some studies suggest that the kinetics of the response were not impacted.[27] For example, in one study, individuals with more severe disease had higher Nab titers than individuals with milder forms of disease but the number of days to peak neutralization titers did not differ based on disease severity.[27] Although Nab titers plateau within a few weeks, Nab titers may be detectable for months.[20] The humoral response in the context of SARS-CoV-2 has been reviewed by multiple groups[5,8,17,28]

Antibody durability has also been studied in response to vaccination. Although there was a slight decline over time, both binding and Nabs were detectable and remained elevated at least 6-months postvaccination with the Moderna vaccine.[29] Postvaccine studies for the Pfizer vaccine yielded similar results, demonstrating sustained antibody durability at least in response to mRNA vaccines. Studies are ongoing to determine when antibodies wane to levels that may warrant a booster dose of these vaccines.

In conclusion, individuals who are infected with SARS-CoV-2 and are symptomatic develop SARS-CoV-2 specific antibodies. IgM rises quickly and peaks 2 to 5-weeks postsymptom onset and then rapidly declines to undetectable levels within another 3 to 5 weeks. In contrast, IgG peaks 3 to 7-week postdisease onset, then plateaus and moderately declines for the next few weeks but can persist and be detected for several months postinfection.[20,22] Because there is no significant delay between IgM and IgG seroconversion, serology should not be used to diagnose SARS-CoV-2 infection, and there is no substantial benefit for using IgM standalone assays. In addition, for assessing exposure weeks after symptom onset IgG is useful as it is more durable. Vaccine-induced antibodies are detectable at least 6-months postvaccine administration of either of the 2 mRNA vaccines, Moderna and Pfizer.[14,30] Ongoing studies will further refine these findings.

SEVERE ACUTE RESPIRATORY SYNDROME CORONAVIRUS 2 SEROLOGY TESTING LANDSCAPE

As of April 2021, the FDA site lists 75 serology assays that have received EUA in the United States. Currently available commercial serology assays vary in methodology, antibody class detection, and antigen targets. There are 3 general types of methodologies: ELISA, LFA that provide rapid results and chemiluminescent immunoassays (CIA) Often, an individual major manufacturer may have multiple assays that have received EUA. For example, a single manufacturer may have an IgG, an IgM, and a total antibody assay. In addition, some vendors also have the same antibody class for a different target, such as a nucleocapsid IgG assay and a spike IgG assay. A few assays detect antibodies to more than one viral protein target. The vast majority of the assays are approved for use in high and moderate complexity settings. Only 5 of the many rapid, LFA are CLIA-waived. Sample types include plasma and serum, fingerstick whole blood, and the most recent addition, dried blood spot for home collection. Only a handful of the assays are semiquantitative, and one has EUA claim for specifically detecting Nabs. The following link (https://www.fda.gov/medical-devices/coronavirus-disease-2019-covid-19-emergency-use-authorizations-medical-devices/in-vitro-diagnostics-euas-serology-and-other-adaptive-immune-response-tests-sars-cov-2) to the FDA site is a helpful reference as it lists the current EUA serology assays available and general overview of the assay. Another useful link is: https://www.fda.gov/medical-devices/coronavirus-disease-2019-covid-19-emergency-use-authorizations-medical-devices/eua-authorized-serology-test-performance. At this site, one can not only read the instructions for use (IFU), instructions for health care providers and test recipients for each assay but can also quickly ascertain the performance characteristics of a serology assay based on the data the manufacturer provided and additional findings if the assay was independently evaluated by NCI, CDC, or BARDA. Needless to say, the sheer number of serology assay options for a single infectious agent is not only unprecedented but makes navigating the testing landscape increasingly difficult.

SEVERE ACUTE RESPIRATORY SYNDROME CORONAVIRUS 2 SEROLOGY ASSAY DESIGNS
Binding Antibody Assays

The vast majority of commercial assays are geared toward detecting the IgG isotype, but there are several total antibody assays, IgM & IgG combination (particularly for LFA), and a few IgM standalone assays that have received EUA. Although IgA assays have been developed, they are not in use in the United States, as studies have shown that they lack specificity. Professional guidelines do not recommend IgA assays or the use of a standalone IgM assay but do not otherwise express a preference for assays based on antibody class(es) detected.[15,16,31] IgG and total antibody assays have become the most commonly used assays because antibody testing is not recommended for diagnosis. Therefore, assays that detect IgG or total antibodies can be used to determine exposure and are the most widely used.

Antibody isotype is just one of the SARS-CoV-2 serology assay attributes that a laboratory must consider when choosing which SARS-CoV-2 assay to implement. Another important consideration is the viral target of the assay. SARS-CoV-2 consists of a single-stranded positive-sense RNA genome which encodes for nonstructural and 4 structural proteins, including the spike (S) and the nucleocapsid (N) proteins. The spike glycoprotein, S1 subunit is a surface protein present on the virion that contains the RBD which binds the angiotensin-converting enzyme 2 (ACE2) receptor and mediates entry into the host cell. The RBD and spike protein are the primary targets for Nabs in SARS-CoV-2 infection. Nabs prevent viral infection of the cell by interfering with the ability of the virus to interact with the ACE2 cell surface receptor.[32,33] Assays may contain different spike regions as targets, including S1 & S2, S1 only, or RBD only. The N protein is the most abundantly expressed viral protein and encapsulates viral RNA. It is well established that antibody responses against the nucleocapsid and spike proteins of the SARS-CoV-2 virus are readily detected in individuals who have been infected with SARS-CoV-2 and have also become the favored targets for serology assays.[25] There are some assays that use both the S and N proteins as antigenic targets.[4,34,35] Although both of these targets have been used extensively in developing serology assays for determining exposure to SARS-CoV-2, recent attention has turned to IgG antibody assays against the spike protein, as a possible tool for assessing immune response due to vaccination.

Severe Acute Respiratory Syndrome Coronavirus 2 Nab Assays

Although Nabs play a crucial role in SARS-CoV-2 infection, there is only one assay that has received EUA that specifically detects Nabs. This is in part because developing a Nab assay that can be adapted to a clinical laboratory is difficult to achieve. The gold standard for measuring Nabs is the plaque reduction neutralization test (PRNT). A classic PRNT assay determines the serum dilution that inhibits viral growth (50% or 90% inhibition) in cell culture and can therefore provide a titer. However, these assays require expertise in cell culture, are labor-intensive and require live virus, which in the case of SARS-CoV-2 would necessitate a biosafety level 3 (BSL3) facility. Another methodology is the pseudovirus-based live cell neutralization assay. This methodology uses a pseudoviral vector to express the protein target of interest, such as the spike for SARS-CoV-2, therefore eliminating the need for live SARS-CoV-2 virus and a BSL3 facility. However, this method still requires viral and cell culture expertise and is not amenable to high throughput settings and rapid turnaround time (TAT), as needed for implementation in a clinical laboratory. These classical methods that use live or pseudotyped virus and determine the serum dilution that inhibits virus growth maybe the gold standard for measuring Nab concentrations but are really only suited for research.[24,36–38] More recently, surrogate viral neutralization tests (sVNT) have been developed. sVNT have a percent inhibition cut-off that allows for a qualitative determination of presence or absence of Nabs.[39] The Nab assay that has received EUA uses the spike protein as a target because the primary target of Nabs is the spike protein. The assay does not detect a particular antibody class. The role of Nab assays in the clinical laboratory remains to be determined.

EVALUATION OF SEVERE ACUTE RESPIRATORY SYNDROME CORONAVIRUS 2 SEROLOGY ASSAYS

As mentioned above, the FDA now requires that manufacturers of SARS-CoV-2 antibody assays submit supporting data to FDA within 10 days of notifying the FDA of the intent to bring an antibody assay to market and has published specific templates with sample size and performance threshold recommendations for EUA submission for serology assays. Although there are many caveats in the template depending on whether the assay is designed to detect individual or combined SARS-CoV-2 antibody classes, there are some general rules. Evaluation of at least 75 unique samples, preferably collected from subjects before December 2020, is recommended for specificity studies. Furthermore, if the 75 samples were tested from a population that has a high prevalence of vaccination against, and/or infection with common viruses and the observed percent positive agreement (PPA) is greater than 95% then specific cross-reactivity studies are not required. Evaluation of sensitivity requires a minimum of 30 unique samples collected from individuals with RT-PCR confirmed SARS-CoV-2 infection. Clinical performance data for sensitivity is stratified by days postsymptom onset and the typical timeframes suggested are 0 to 7 days, 8 to 14 days, and $\geq$ 15 days. For IgG and total antibody assays, 30 samples collected at day 15 or later postsymptom onset, are recommended. Therefore, for SARS-CoV-2 serology assays, generally, the minimum PPA required is 90% and the minimum negative percent agreement is 95%.[40]

SEVERE ACUTE RESPIRATORY SYNDROME CORONAVIRUS 2 SEROLOGY TESTING RECOMMENDATIONS

SARS-CoV-2 serology testing is recommended by a number of professional societies for the following applications: (1) seroprevalence and epidemiologic studies, (2) as an aid in diagnosing multisystem inflammatory syndrome in children (MIS-C), (3) support a diagnosis in individuals with symptoms consistent with SARS-CoV-2 infection who repeatedly test negative by NAAT, and (4) identifying eligible COVID-19 convalescent plasma (CCP) donors.

Serology assays have been used extensively for seroprevalence studies.[41] Given that a large proportion of adults have now been immunized in the United States, serology-based seroprevalence studies are more difficult to interpret. Careful consideration must be given to the choice of the assay and respective antigenic target used for this type of investigation (please see below).

Serologic testing can also be helpful clinically for the diagnosis of both MIS-C and adults who present late in the disease course. MIS-C develops in some children infected with SARS-CoV-2, often after the viral infection is no longer detectable by NAAT.[42] Serology testing for MIS-C is now a criterion included in the case definition..[31] For adults who have symptoms consistent with SARS-CoV-2 infection or have been exposed to SARS-CoV-2 infection but are repeatedly NAAT negative, antibody testing can also be used as the confirmation of SARS-CoV-2 infection. Generally, the use of either an IgG or a total antibody assay at 3 to 4 weeks (no sooner than 14 days) post-symptom onset for optimal accuracy, when using serology assays as an adjunct for the confirmation of SARS-CoV-2 infection is recommended.[15,31,34]

The use of convalescent plasma to treat patients with COVID-19 was implemented early during the pandemic. Passive antibody transfer as a therapy has been used for a number of infectious diseases in the past, including influenza.[43] Initially, only one commercial assay was approved for the selection of individuals considered to have "high SARS-CoV-2 antibody titers" and who were eligible for COVID-19 convalescent donations. However, in recent months, the FDA has updated the guidelines and has now established individual manufacturer-dependent cut-offs for several commercial assays that measure binding antibodies that can be used for the qualification of high antibody titer samples that can be used for CCP donations.

One serology testing application that has been used in the research setting but has yet to be used clinically, is to monitor vaccine response. As of May 2021, there are no recommendations for determining who should qualify for vaccination or what is considered an appropriate or protective immune response postvaccine administration based on serology results.[16] This is due to both the way vaccine efficacy was assessed during the vaccine clinical trials and the lack of standardization for both binding and Nab assays. Vaccine trials evaluated vaccine efficacy by comparing how many individuals became infected with SARS-CoV-2 in the control and vaccinated groups during the course of the clinical trials. And although various binding and Nab assays were used to determine if individuals mounted an immune response there was no cut-off on any assay that was evaluated for protective immunity.[14] In fact, 100% of vaccinated individuals developed robust levels of binding and Nabs in response to vaccination with the Moderna mRNA vaccine.[14] Although currently there are no recommendations for monitoring or assessing appropriate immune response due to vaccination using serology testing, many individuals who have been vaccinated have sought serology testing postvaccination. And although a detectable immune response postvaccination indicates that the individual has mounted an immune response to the vaccination, it is imperative to emphasize that there is no threshold antibody level associated with protective immunity on any platform, including Nab assays.

SEVERE ACUTE RESPIRATORY SYNDROME CORONAVIRUS 2 SEROLOGY TEST REPORTING AND INTERPRETATION

SARS-CoV-2 antibody test result interpretation is complex. Although in its simplest form, a negative antibody result indicates no SARS-CoV-2 exposure or vaccination, and a positive antibody result suggests exposure or possibly vaccination, all results must be interpreted in context. Variables that impact interpretation include: timing of the sample collection, patient clinical history, antigen target, and performance characteristics of the assay used.

Timing of sample collection in serology testing is crucial for appropriate test interpretation. Most notably, suboptimal timing due to the early collection of sample postsymptom onset can result in a false-negative result. A false-negative result in someone who was exposed to SARS-CoV-2 is also possible in patients who are immunocompromised or individuals who had asymptomatic infection.[44]

Antigenic targets further complicate the interpretation. Due to the mass vaccination success in the United States, the antigen target has become a recent conundrum. Clinicians and epidemiologists may want to determine who has been exposed to infection and who has been vaccinated. Because the spike protein is the target of the vaccines that have been approved to date in the United States, it is reasonable to think that one can distinguish between these 2 scenarios by testing for spike and nucleocapsid antibodies. For example, individuals who are positive by nucleocapsid assays must have had a natural infection because the vaccines do not use nucleocapsid as the antigen for antibody stimulation. Indeed most recent updates from the CDC reflect this approach and test interpretation.[16] However, caution must be taken because, in the absence of clinical history, this approach is predicated on the assumption that the nucleocapsid and spike assays used in a laboratory have the same sensitivity and specificity which is not likely. There have been reports of known, confirmed SARS-COV-2 cases that subsequently tested positive by a spike assay but negative by a nucleocapsid assay.[45,46] Clinical history is crucial to correct test result interpretation, otherwise, test results could translate in misclassifying an individual's status. Seroprevalence studies and reference laboratories may be particularly challenged by the lack of clinical history to assist in test interpretation. The merits of using nucleocapsid and spike assays to distinguish between vaccinated and previously infected individuals is an active area of research and publications are forthcoming.[47]

In addition, assay performance characteristics not only vary between assays, but even small differences in specificity and sensitivity between assays can translate to substantial differences in positive predictive value (PPV) and negative predictive value (NPV) depending on disease prevalence. For example, an assay that has 98.1% sensitivity and 99.6% specificity that translates into 99.9% NPV and only 92% PPV when disease prevalence is 5.0%. If the disease prevalence is 10% the NPV only drops to 99.8% but the PPV increases to 96.1%. It is understandable that PPV was of particular concern during the early days of the pandemic, when disease prevalence was low. Therefore, the CDC made the following recommendation to increase PPV: (1) test only individuals who have a high likelihood of exposure to SARS-CoV-2, (2) test with an assay that has greater than 99.5% specificity, and (3) if not possible to test with an assay that has greater than 99.5% specificity then implement an orthogonal approach to testing.[16]

The orthogonal approach to testing is based on testing with one serology assay and if the sample is positive by the first assay, then the sample is tested by a second assay. Ideally, the assay with the highest specificity should be used first to minimize discrepant results between the 2 assays used in an orthogonal testing approach. Otherwise, the assays used in this type of algorithm can be the same antigenic target but different method (ELISA spike and CIA spike), or the same method but different antigenic targets (CIA nucleocapsid, CIA spike). If both test results are positive, then the PPV is very high, assuring that the result is a true positive. However, if the second test is negative interpretation is less clear. Although at first glance this would suggest a false-positive result with the first assay, it may be that the discrepant results are due to differences in sensitivity between the assays and not a reflection of the accuracy of the first test. Discrepant results must be interpreted with caution and considered in the context of the patient's clinical history. Orthogonal testing has also been applied for seroprevalence studies.[41] Today, the prevalence of disease has increased across the country and assays with greater than 99.5% specificity are more readily available;

therefore, the need for orthogonal testing to increase PPV is no longer a priority for most laboratories.

In summary, many variables, including patient history, have an impact on the accuracy of the test result and interpretation. Both the FDA and best practices require that clinical serology results must be accompanied by clear footnotes on the patient chart that state the limitations of serology testing. Most, importantly, serology testing should not be used for diagnosing SARS-CoV-2 infection. Other important limitations include that a negative SARS-CoV-2 antibody result does not rule out current or past infection and a positive SARS-CoV-2 antibody test can be due to cross-reaction with other commonly circulating human coronaviruses. The clearer and more comprehensive yet concise information a laboratory can provide in the test order recommendations and/or chart comments regarding the details of the assay used (such as the antigenic target, antibody class detected) and specific limitations, the more helpful it is for clients, clinicians, and patients.

SEVERE ACUTE RESPIRATORY SYNDROME CORONAVIRUS 2 ANTIBODY TESTING PERSPECTIVE

Although many studies have been conducted to address immunity postinfection and postvaccination, some aspects of humoral immunity in response to SARS-CoV-2 infection are still being defined. Studies have often yielded conflicting results about various aspects of SARS-CoV-2 infection humoral response. It is important to note that many of the studies, particularly early in the pandemic, were limited in patient numbers, patient demographics, and temporal follow-up. More recent studies have had access to larger and more diverse cohorts and extended study duration. Another complicating factor that can affect the result of studies attempting to address the fundamental serology questions in the context of SARS-CoV-2 infection is that the assay used for these studies may also have an impact on the findings. Fundamentally, it is still not known what constitutes a protective immune response when assessing antibody response, in the context of natural infection or vaccination.

Another challenge to making a meaningful interpretation for SARS-CoV-2 antibody test results is the lack of standardization for both binding and Nab assays. Substantial test performance variation and therefore choice of assay can have a significant impact on the overall conclusion of a study or clinical test interpretation.

The lack of standardization between any of the EUA serology assays, neutralizing, and binding antibody assays makes it difficult to interpret results obtained with different serology assays. This is the case for both clinical interpretation and a confounding factor in research studies. Semiquantitative assay results have no commutability and cannot be used interchangeably between assays, even if the assays are semiquantitative. Although the need for standardization is undeniable, the first step is to determine what constitutes humoral protective immunity. Antibodies as a correlate of protective immunity and accompanying standard threshold have been developed for other infectious diseases such as hepatitis B, whereby hepatitis B surface antibody levels more than 10 mIU/mL indicate protective immunity.[43] It is, therefore, possible that someday there will be SARS-CoV-2 antibody manufacturer-specific cut-offs, as has been established for SARS-CoV-2 antibody assays in the context of CCP, or a standard that can be used to firmly establish what constitutes a protective antibody response in the context of SARS-CoV-2.

In summary, the SARS-CoV-2 pandemic continues to dominate the world and US health care. Laboratory testing, including serology testing, remains at the forefront of the public health response. Current antibody testing is not limited by technology or supply chain issues, but important limitations do exist. The limitations consist of rapidly changing understanding of the immune response to natural infection with SARS-CoV-2, evolving knowledge regarding vaccine response to a new form of vaccine technology, and the lack of standardization for serology assays. Although antibody tests are widely available, there is a need for standardization to increase the clinical utility of antibody testing in the future.

The laboratory must remain vigilant in staying current with advancing knowledge, rapid developments in testing methods, and updated recommendations. The laboratory remains critical to ensuring a quality result by validating/verifying the test and implementing appropriate quality control measures.[15] Finally, the laboratory is crucial to educating clinicians, patients, and the public alike about the complexity and limitations of SARS-CoV-2 antibody testing.

CLINICS CARE POINTS

- SARS CoV-2 serology assays are not standardized.
- Clinical utility remains limited.
- If a serology assay is used as an adjunct to nucleic acid amplification tests (NAATs) for supporting a clinical diagnosis in MIS-C or in adults with suspicion of SARS-CoV-2 who are NAAT negative, IgG, and total antibody assays should be used 3 to 4 weeks postsymptom onset for optimal accuracy.

DISCLOSURE

The author has nothing to disclose.

REFERENCES

1. Wu F, Zhao S, Yu B, et al. A new coronavirus associated with human respiratory disease in China. Nature 2020;579(7798):265–9.
2. Theel ES, Slev P, Wheeler S, et al. The role of antibody testing for SARS-CoV-2: is there one? J Clin Microbiol 2020;58(8). e00797-20.
3. Farnsworth CW, Anderson NW. SARS-CoV-2 serology: much hype, little data. Clin Chem 2020;66(7):875–7.
4. Ravi N, Cortade DL, Ng E, et al. Diagnostics for SARS-CoV-2 detection: a comprehensive review of the FDA-EUA COVID-19 testing landscape. Biosens Bioelectron 2020;165:112454.
5. Carrillo J, Izquierdo-Useros N, Avila-Nieto C, et al. Humoral immune responses and neutralizing antibodies against SARS-CoV-2; implications in pathogenesis and protective immunity. Biochem Biophys Res Commun 2021;538:187–91.
6. Zhao J, Yuan Q, Wang H, et al. Antibody responses to SARS-CoV-2 in patients with novel coronavirus disease 2019. Clin Infect Dis 2020;71(16):2027–34.
7. Chi X, Yan R, Zhang J, et al. A neutralizing human antibody binds to the N-terminal domain of the Spike protein of SARS-CoV-2. Science 2020;369(6504):650–5.
8. Hueston L, Kok J, Guibone, et al. The antibody response to SARS-CoV-2 infection. Infectious Diseases Society of merica; 2020. p. 1–8. https://doi.org/10.1093/ofid/ofaa387.
9. Ju B, Zhang Q, Ge J, et al. Human neutralizing antibodies elicited by SARS-CoV-2 infection. Nature 2020;584(7819):115–9.

10. Liu L, Wang P, Nair MS, et al. Potent neutralizing antibodies against multiple epitopes on SARS-CoV-2 spike. Nature 2020;584(7821):450–6.

11. Suhandynata RT, Bevins NJ, Tran JT, et al. SARS-CoV-2 serology status detected by commercialized platforms distinguishes previous infection and vaccination adaptive immune responses. medRxiv : the preprint server for health sciences. medRxiv 2021. https://doi.org/10.1101/2021.03.10.21253299.

12. Liu W, Liu L, Kou G, et al. Evaluation of nucleocapsid and spike protein-based enzyme-linked immunosorbent assays for detecting antibodies against SARS-CoV-2. J Clin Microbiol 2020;58(6). e00461-20.

13. Rychert J, Couturier MR, Elgort M, et al. Evaluation of 3 SARS-CoV-2 IgG antibody assays and correlation with neutralizing antibodies. J Appl Lab Med 2021;6(3):614–24.

14. Jackson LA, Anderson EJ, Rouphael NG, et al. An mRNA vaccine against SARS-CoV-2 - preliminary report. N Engl J Med 2020;383(20):1920–31.

15. Zhang YV, Wiencek J, Meng QH, et al. AACC practical recommendations for implementing and interpreting SARS-CoV-2 EUA and LDT Serologic Testing in Clinical Laboratories. Clin Chem 2021;67(9):1188–200.

16. CDC. Interim guidelines for COVID-19 antibody testing. Available at: https://www.cdc.gov/coronavirus/2019-ncov/lab/resources/antibody-tests-guidelines.html. Accessed May 20, 2021.

17. Post N, Eddy D, Huntley C, et al. Antibody response to SARS-CoV-2 infection in humans: a systematic review. PLoS One 2020;15(12):e0244126.

18. Long QX, Liu BZ, Deng HJ, et al. Antibody responses to SARS-CoV-2 in patients with COVID-19. Nat Med 2020;26(6):845–8.

19. Long QX, Tang XJ, Shi QL, et al. Clinical and immunological assessment of asymptomatic SARS-CoV-2 infections. Nat Med 2020;26(8):1200–4.

20. Wajnberg A, Amanat F, Firpo A, et al. Robust neutralizing antibodies to SARS-CoV-2 infection persist for months. Science 2020;370(6521):1227–30.

21. Dan JM, Mateus J, Kato Y, et al. Immunological memory to SARS-CoV-2 assessed for up to 8 months after infection. Science 2021;371(6529). eabf4063.

22. Gudbjartsson DF, Norddahl GL, Melsted P, et al. Humoral immune response to SARS-CoV-2 in Iceland. N Engl J Med 2020;383(18):1724–34.

23. Wang P, Liu L, Nair MS, et al. SARS-CoV-2 neutralizing antibody responses are more robust in patients with severe disease. Emerg Microbes Infect 2020;9(1):2091–3.

24. Wu F, Liu M, Wang A, et al. Evaluating the association of clinical characteristics with neutralizing antibody levels in patients who have recovered from mild COVID-19 in shanghai, China. JAMA Intern Med 2020;180(10):1356–62.

25. Shrock E, Fujimura E, Kula T, et al. Viral epitope profiling of COVID-19 patients reveals cross-reactivity and correlates of severity. Science 2020;370(6520). eabd4250.

26. Wang K, Long QX, Deng HJ, et al. Longitudinal dynamics of the neutralizing antibody response to SARS-CoV-2 infection. Clin Infect Dis 2021 Aug 2;73(3):e531–9.

27. Seow J, Graham C, Merrick B, et al. Longitudinal observation and decline of neutralizing antibody responses in the three months following SARS-CoV-2 infection in humans. Nat Microbiol. 2020 Dec;12(5):1598–607.

28. Vabret N, Britton GJ, Gruber C, et al. Immunology of COVID-19: current state of the science. Immunity 2020;52(6):910–41.

29. Doria-Rose N, Suthar MS, Makowski M, et al. Antibody persistence through 6 Months after the second dose of mRNA-1273 vaccine for covid-19. N Engl J Med 2021;384(23):2259–61.

30. pfizer. PFIZER AND BIONTECH CONFIRM HIGH EFFICACY AND NO SERIOUS SAFETY CONCERNS THROUGH UP TO SIX MONTHS FOLLOWING SECOND DOSE IN UPDATED TOPLINE ANALYSIS OF LANDMARK COVID-19 VACCINE STUDY. 2021. Available at: https://www.pfizer.com/news/press-release/press-release-detail/pfizer-and-biontech-confirm-high-efficacy-and-no-serious#:%7E:text=19%20Vaccine%20Study-,PFIZER%20AND%20BIONTECH%20CONFIRM%20HIGH%20EFFICACY%20AND%20NO%20SERIOUS%20SAFETY%20CONCERNS%20THROUGH%20UP%20. Accessed May 20, 2021.

31. Hanson KE, Caliendo AM, Arias CA, et al. Infectious diseases society of America guidelines on the diagnosis of COVID-19:serologic testing. Clin Infect Dis 2020. https://doi.org/10.1093/cid/ciaa1343.

32. Walls AC, Park YJ, Tortorici MA, et al. Structure, function, and Antigenicity of the SARS-CoV-2 spike glycoprotein. Cell 2020;181(2):281–92.e6.

33. Wu Y, Wang F, Shen C, et al. A noncompeting pair of human neutralizing antibodies block COVID-19 virus binding to its receptor ACE2. Science 2020;368(6496):1274–8.

34. Deeks JJ, Dinnes J, Takwoingi Y, et al. Antibody tests for identification of current and past infection with SARS-CoV-2. Cochrane Database Syst Rev 2020;6:CD013652.

35. Lisboa Bastos M, Tavaziva G, Abidi SK, et al. Diagnostic accuracy of serological tests for covid-19: systematic review and meta-analysis. Bmj 2020;370:m2516.

36. Zheng Y, Larragoite ET, Lama J, et al. Neutralization assay with SARS-CoV-1 and SARS-CoV-2 spike pseudotyped murine leukemia virions. bioRxiv 2020. https://doi.org/10.1101/2020.07.17.207563.

37. Amanat F, Stadlbauer D, Strohmeier S, et al. A serological assay to detect SARS-CoV-2 seroconversion in humans. Nat Med 2020;26(7):1033–6.

38. Okba NMA, Müller MA, Li W, et al. Severe acute respiratory syndrome coronavirus 2-specific antibody responses in coronavirus disease patients. Emerg Infect Dis 2020;26(7):1478–88.

39. Tan CW, Chia WN, Qin X, et al. A SARS-CoV-2 surrogate virus neutralization test based on antibody-mediated blockage of ACE2-spike protein-protein interaction. Nat Biotechnol 2020;38(9):1073–8.

40. (FDA) UFaDA. Serology template for test developers. Available at: https://www.fda.gov/medical-devices/coronavirus-disease-2019-covid-19-emergency-use-authorizations-medical-devices/in-vitro-diagnostics-euas. Accessed May 20, 2021.

41. Ripperger TJ, Uhrlaub JL, Watanabe M, et al. Orthogonal SARS-CoV-2 serological assays enable surveillance of low-prevalence communities and reveal durable humoral immunity. Immunity 2020;53(5):925–33.e4.

42. Whittaker E, Bamford A, Kenny J, et al. Clinical characteristics of 58 children with a pediatric inflammatory multisystem syndrome temporally associated with SARS-CoV-2. JAMA 2020;324(3):259–69.

43. Plotkin SA. Updates on immunologic correlates of vaccine-induced protection. Vaccine 2020;38(9):2250–7.

44. Ye X, Xiao X, Li B, et al. Low humoral immune response and ineffective clearance of SARS-cov-2 in a COVID-19 patient with CLL during a 69-day follow-up. Front Oncol 2020;10:1272.

45. Wang H, Wiredja D, Yang L, et al. Case-control study of individuals with discrepant nucleocapsid and spike protein SARS-CoV-2 IgG results. Clin Chem 2021;67(7):977–86.
46. Röltgen K, Powell AE, Wirz OF, et al. Defining the features and duration of antibody responses to SARS-CoV-2 infection associated with disease severity and outcome. Sci Immunol 2020;5(54). eabe0240.
47. Demmer RT, Baumgartner B, Wiggen TD, et al. Identification of natural SARS-CoV-2 infection in seroprevalence studies among vaccinated populations. medRxiv 2021. https://doi.org/10.1101/2021.04.12.21255330.

Performance Characteristics of High-Throughput Serologic Assays for Severe Acute Respiratory Syndrome Coronavirus 2 with Food and Drug Administration Emergency Use Authorization: A Review

Elitza S. Theel, PhD, D(ABMM)

KEYWORDS

- SARS-CoV-2 • COVID-19 • Antibody • Serology • High-throughput assays

KEY POINTS

- The currently available high-throughput severe acute respiratory syndrome coronavirus 2 (SARS-CoV-2) serologic assays with Food and Drug Administration (FDA) Emergency Use Authorization (EUA) are quite heterogeneous, detecting different antibody classes (eg, immunoglobulin M (IgM), IgG, total immunoglobulin) against a variety of SARS-CoV-2 antigens (eg, spike glycoprotein, receptor-binding domain) using a variety of different methods (eg, enzyme-linked immunosorbent assays, chemiluminescent immunoassays, and so forth). Understanding the advantages, limitations, and performance characteristics of each is necessary before implementation in the clinical laboratory.
- Serologic assays with high specificity (ie, ≥99.5%) are preferred in low disease prevalence settings to maximize the positive predictive value of serologic test results. Most of the SARS-CoV-2 serologic assays with FDA EUA have documented specificity ranges approaching 100% among prepandemic and cross-reactivity panels.
- The sensitivity of SARS-CoV-2 serologic assays is affected by multiple factors, including disease severity, patient immunostatus, and timing of sample collection postsymptom onset, among others. Most of the patients with COVID-19 are seropositive after at least 14 days of symptoms.

Division of Clinical Microbiology, Department of Laboratory Medicine and Pathology, Mayo Clinic, Room 1-526, 3050 Superior Drive Northwest, Rochester, MN 55901, USA
E-mail address: theel.elitza@mayo.edu
Twitter: @ElliTheelPhD (E.S.T.)

Clin Lab Med 42 (2022) 15–29
https://doi.org/10.1016/j.cll.2021.10.006
0272-2712/22/© 2021 Elsevier Inc. All rights reserved.

INTRODUCTION

Throughout the coronavirus disease 2019 (COVID-19) pandemic, the role of serologic testing for severe acute respiratory syndrome coronavirus 2 (SARS-CoV-2) has been debated among clinicians and laboratorians. In contrast, among both public and government forums, interest in this methodology has oscillated between "none," to headlines suggesting that such testing may help to "reopen economies."[1,2] In reality, the truth lies somewhere in between these 2 dichotomies. Currently, the role of serologic testing for SARS-CoV-2 in the clinical realm remains fairly limited and of note, has not significantly changed since the start of the pandemic. These potential uses, not solely limited to the clinical setting, include the following[3–5]:

- Aid in the diagnosis of COVID-19 in patients with a negative SARS-CoV-2 molecular or antigen detection assay, who present at least 7 days after disease onset and with a prior negative antibody test result
- Aid in the diagnosis of complications associated with COVID-19, including multisystem inflammatory syndrome in children
- Manufacture of COVID-19 convalescent plasma
- Use for SARS-CoV-2 seroprevalence surveys to document incidence of natural infection and/or vaccination
- Use in research (eg, vaccine efficacy, immunity, humoral immune response kinetics, and so forth)

As with any emerging pathogen, the development and deployment of clinical laboratory methods for the detection of SARS-CoV-2, including molecular, antigenic, and serologic tests, occurred in parallel to our growing understanding of virus' pathology and optimal test utilization practices. With respect to serologic methods specifically, more than 200 assays were commercially available in the United States early in the pandemic due to multiple factors, including high consumer interest and limited oversight from the US Food and Drug Administration (FDA), which did not require Emergence Use Authorization (EUA) for SARS-CoV-2 serologic assays, unlike for molecular and antigenic assays, until May 4th, 2020.[6] As of the writing of this article (April 2021), there are currently 75 SARS-CoV-2 serologic assays with FDA EUA, and more than 260 assays that the FDA specifically indicates should not be used or distributed due to either poor performance, lack of EUA receipt, or voluntary removal from the market by the manufacturer.[7]

Among the SARS-CoV-2 serologic tests with FDA EUA, there is significant variability in the methods (eg, enzyme linked immunosorbent assays [ELISAs], chemiluminescent immunoassays [CIAs], lateral flow immunoassays, and so forth.) and design characteristics (eg, SARS-CoV-2 antigen used, targeted antibody class, result reporting, and so forth.) of these assays, which may affect their clinical performance characteristics, sample throughput, and the capability of laboratories to implement them in their local facility settings. This article focuses on discussing the performance characteristics of commonly used high-throughput assays with FDA EUA for detection of SARS-CoV-2 antibodies in the central clinical laboratory. For a discussion of lateral flow assays or alternative means for detection of antibodies to SARS-CoV-2, the reader is referred to Ochola and colleagues' article, "Performance Evaluation of Lateral Flow Assays for COVID-19 Serology," and Patel and colleagues' article, "Alternative Methods to Detect SARS-CoV-2 Antibodies," in this issue.

Table 1
Summary of select high-throughput, automated serologic assays with FDA EUA for detection of antibodies to SARS-CoV-2

Assay Name (Manufacturer)	Method	Antibody Class Detected	SARS-CoV-2 Antigen	Platform/Analyzer	Result Output	FDA-Reported Sensitivity[b] (95% CI)	FDA-Reported Specificity[b] (95% CI)
AdviseDx SARS-CoV-2 IgM (Abbott Laboratories Inc.)	CMIA	IgM	S	Architect i or Alinity i	Qualitative	95% (89.9%–100%)	99.6% (94.6%–99.8%)
AdviseDx SARS-CoV-2 IgG II (Abbott Laboratories Inc.)	CMIA	IgG	RBD	Architect i or Alinity i	Semiquantitative	NA	NA
SARS-CoV-2 IgG Assay (Abbott Laboratories Inc.)	CMIA	IgG	NC	Architect i or Alinity i	Qualitative	100% (89.9%–100%)	≥ 99% (94%–99.8%)
Access SARS-CoV-2 IgG (Beckman Coulter, Inc.)	CIA	IgG	RBD	Access 2, Dxl 600, Dxl 800	Qualitative	96.8% (91.1%–98.9%)	99.6% (99.2%–99.8%)
Access SARS-CoV-2 IgM (Beckman Coulter, Inc.)	CIA	IgM	RBD	Access 2, Dxl 600, Dxl 800	Qualitative	96.7% (92.5%–98.6%)	99.9% (99.5%–100%)
Access SARS-CoV-2 IgG II (Beckman Coulter, Inc.)	CIA	IgG	RBD	Access 2, Dxl 600, Dxl 800	Semiquantitative	NA	NA
Platelia SARS-CoV-2 Total Ab (Bio-Rad Laboratories Inc.)	ELISA	Total	NC	Microplate washer/reader[a]	Qualitative	98% (89.5%–99.6%)	99.3% (98.3%–99.7%)
VIDAS SARS-CoV-2 IgM (bioMerieux SA)	ELFA	IgM	RBD	VIDAS, MINI VIDAS, VIDAS 3	Qualitative	100% (85.7%–100%)	99.4% (97.7%–99.8%)
VIDAS SARS-CoV-2 IgG (bioMerieux SA)	ELFA	IgG	RBD	VIDAS, MINI VIDAS, VIDAS 3	Qualitative	100% (88.3%–100%)	99.9% (99.4%–100%)

(continued on next page)

Table 1
(continued)

Assay Name (Manufacturer)	Method	Antibody Class Detected	SARS-CoV-2 Antigen	Platform/Analyzer	Result Output	FDA-Reported Sensitivity[b] (95% CI)	FDA-Reported Specificity[b] (95% CI)
LIAISON SARS-CoV-2 S1/s2 IgG (DiaSorin Inc.)	CIA	IgG	S1/s2	LIAISON XL	Qualitative	97.6% (87.4%–99.6%)	99.3% (98.6%–99.6%)
LISAISON SARS_CoV-2 IgM (DiaSorin Inc.)	Indirect CIA	IgM	RBD	LIAISON XL	Qualitative	91.8% (85.6%–95.5%)	99.3% (98.9%–99.5%)
Anti-SARS-CoV-2 ELISA (IgG) (EUROIMMUN US Inc.)	ELISA	IgG	S1	Microplate washer/reader[a]	Qualitative	90% (74.4%–96.5%)	100% (95.4%–100%)
cPass SARS-CoV-2 Neutralization Antibody Detection Kit (GenScript USA Inc)	Blocking ELISA	nAb	RBD	Microplate washer/reader[a]	Qualitative	100% (87.1%–100%)	100% (95.8%–100%)
SCoV-2 Detect IgG ELISA (InBios International Inc.)	ELISA	IgG	Not Indicated	Microplate washer/reader[a]	Qualitative	100% (88.7%–100%)	100% (95.4%–100%)
SCoV-2 Detect IgM ELISA (InBios International Inc.)	ELISA	IgM	Not indicated	Microplate washer/reader[a]	Qualitative	96.7% (83.3%–100%)	98.8% (93.3%–100%)
xMAP SARS-CoV-2 Multi-Antigen IgG (Luminex Corp)	FMIA	IgG	S1/RBD/NC	FlexMap 3D, MAGPIX, Luminex 200	Qualitative	96.2% (89.8%–98.7%)	99.3% (98.3%–99.7%)
VITROS Anti-SARS-CoV-2 Total (Ortho Clinical Diagnostics, Inc.)	CIA	Total Ab	S1	VITROS 5600/XT 7600, VITROS ECi/ECiQ/3600	Qualitative	100% (92.7%–100%)	100% (99%–100%)

Assay	Method	Antibody	Antigen	Instrument	Qualitative/Semiquantitative	Sensitivity	Specificity
VITROS Anti-SARS-CoV-2 IgG (Ortho Clinical Diagnostics, Inc.)	CIA	IgG	S	VITROS 5600/XT 7600, VITROS ECi/ECiQ/3600	Qualitative	90% (76.9%–96%)	100% (99.1%–100%)
Elecsys Anti-SARS-CoV-2 (Roche Diagnostics)	ECLIA	Total Ab	NC	cobas e411/e602/e801	Qualitative	100% (88.3%–100%)	99.8% (99.7%–100%)
Elecsys Anti-SARS-CoV-2 s (Roche Diagnostics)	ECLIA	IgG	RBD	cobas e411/e602/e801	Semiquantitative	96.6% (93.4%–98.3%)	100% (99.9%–100%)
SARS-CoV-2 Total (Siemens Healthcare Diagnostics)	CIA	Total Ab	RBD	Atellica IM Analyzer, ADVIA Centaur, Dimension Vista System	Qualitative	100% (91.6%–100%)	99.8% (99.3%–99.9%)
SARS-CoV-2 IgG (Siemens Healthcare Diagnostics)	CIA	IgG	RBD	Atellica IM Analyzer, ADVIA Centaur, Dimension Vista System	Semiquantitative	100% (91.6%–100%)	99.9% (99.6%–100%)
OmniPATH COVID-19 Total Antibody (Thermo Fisher Scientific)	ELISA	Total Ab	RBD	Microplate washer/reader[a] or Dynex Agility	Qualitative	96.7% (83.3%–99.4%)	97.5% (91.3%–99.3%)
SARS-CoV-2 IgG Test System (Zeus Scientific Inc)	ELISA	IgG	RBD/NC	Microplate washer/reader[a]	Qualitative	93.3% (78.7%–98.2%)	100% (94.8%–100%)

Abbreviations: CI, confidence interval; CIA, chemiluminescent immunoassay; CMIA, chemiluminescent microparticle immunoassay; ELFA, enzyme-linked fluorescence assay; ELISA, enzyme-linked immunosorbent assay; FDA, US Food and Drug Administration; FMIA, fluorescent microbead immunoassay; nAb, neutralizing antibody; NC, nucleocapsid; RBD, receptor binding domain; S, spike glycoprotein; S1, spike glycoprotein subunit 1; S2, spike glycoprotein subunit 2.

[a] Laboratories may alternatively validate these on fully automated ELISA processors.

[b] Data from FDA EUA Authorized Serology Test Performance: https://www.fda.gov/medical-devices/coronavirus-disease-2019-covid-19-emergency-use-authorizations-medical-devices/eua-authorized-serology-test-performance.

KEY DESIGN DIFFERENCES AMONG SARS-CoV-2 HIGH-THROUGHPUT SEROLOGIC ASSAYS WITH FDA EUA

Although not an exhaustive list, the more commonly used, automated SARS-CoV-2 serologic assays are listed in **Table 1**, alongside defining method and format characteristics. Most of these assays are based on either chemiluminescent or enzymatic reactions, with fewer assays using fluorescence as the output marker. Although the CIAs and fluorescence-based immunoassays are typically designed to be performed on specific automated platforms, ELISAs may be semiautomated using microplate washers and readers, or may be fully automated using open-system ELISA processors, following completion of laboratory validation/verification studies. In addition, although most of the assays, regardless of format, provide qualitative results only, an increasing number of assays are receiving FDA EUA as semi-quantitative methods, reporting out results in "arbitrary units (AU)" per mL, alongside a qualitative interpretation. Importantly, however, although there is now a SARS-CoV-2 immunoglobulin G (IgG) standard available through the World Health Organization (WHO), widespread standardization among the high-throughput semi-quantitative assays has not yet occurred.[8] Therefore, the reported values are not interchangeable across platforms, and significant variability has been observed between methods.[9,10]

Another key differential feature of serologic assays is the SARS-CoV-2 antigen they are based on, which varies between epitopes of either the viral spike (S) glycoprotein or the nucleocapsid (NC) protein (see **Table 1**). The S glycoprotein decorates the surface of SARS-CoV-2 and mediates binding to and fusion with the human angiotensin-converting enzyme 2 (ACE2) for cellular entry and is also the primary target for neutralizing antibodies to the virus.[11] More specifically, each monomer of the S trimer is composed of 2 subunits—S1 and S2. Within the S1 subunit lies the receptor binding domain (RBD), which specifically interacts with the ACE2 receptor for binding. Most of the high-throughput serologic assays have been designed to detect antibodies to recombinant versions of the RBD, followed by recombinant S or S1 antigens (see **Table 1**). Less frequently, manufacturers have used recombinant SARS-CoV-2 NC as the target antigen, which is also highly immunogenic but is involved with viral RNA replication, packaging, and viral particle release.[12] Although there are some reports suggesting differential sensitivity of serologic assays based on whether SARS-CoV-2 S or NC components are targeted, knowing which antigen the serologic assay is based on is increasingly important from the perspective of result interpretation in the setting of increasing SARS-CoV-2 vaccination rates. Currently, all of the SARS-CoV-2 vaccines with FDA EUA are designed to induce a humoral and cellular immune response to the S glycoprotein.[13] Therefore, although anti-S/RBD/S1/S2-based serologic assays may result as positive in either vaccinated or naturally infected individuals, anti-NC assays will only be positive in those who have had a prior natural infection with SARS-CoV-2.

The final key differential feature among high-throughput SARS-CoV-2 serologic assays is the antibody type and the class or classes of antibodies detected (see **Table 1**). Currently all but one of the serologic assays with FDA EUA detect *binding* antibodies to the virus, with a single assay specifically detecting *neutralizing* antibodies (nAb; cPass GenScript USA Inc.). Although binding antibodies will recognize different immunogenic viral epitopes, their binding antibodies may either not affect infectivity or they may recruit other components of the immune system to help inactivate the virus (eg, via opsonization or complement fixation). In contrast, nAb recognize and specifically bind to viral epitopes involved with cellular entry and replication, resulting in the inhibition of viral infectivity, independent of other elements of the immune system. The presence of nAb has typically been used as a correlate for protective immunity for a variety of infectious diseases and has been shown to increase alongside binding antibodies following both natural infection with and vaccination against SARS-CoV-2.[14–17]

PERFORMANCE CHARACTERISTICS AMONG THE COMMONLY USED HIGH-THROUGHPUT SARS-CoV-2 SEROLOGIC ASSAYS

The selection of which high-throughput SARS-CoV-2 serologic assay to implement in the central laboratory depends on multiple factors beyond just the reported performance of the assay, including factors such as which platforms are available in the laboratory and have excess capacity, reagent cost, and workflow considerations, among others. Following selection, the assay must be verified before clinical use, which early during the pandemic was challenging for multiple reasons, including limited availability of well-characterized specimens, lack of a reference standard method and an unclear understanding of what is required for verification of assays with FDA EUA. In an effort to provide guidance to laboratories both during the current and for future pandemics, multiple organizations, including the American Society for Microbiology and the American Association for Clinical Chemistry, put forth detailed documents for verification of serologic assays with EUA during a pandemic, to which the reader is referred.[18,19]

With the rapid development and deployment of SARS-CoV-2 serologic tests and increasing unease regarding the accuracy associated with several of these assays, the FDA put forth an easily accessible summary of assay-specific performance characteristics, which were used to base the decision for EUA authorization.[20] These data were provided by the assay manufacturer as part of the EUA application process and/or from testing performed at the National Cancer Institute and are summarized in **Table 1**. Overall, sensitivity and specificity values for these assays were high, ranging from 90% to 100% and 97.5% to 100%, respectively. However, these data do not provide a complete picture, as sensitivity can vary depending on time of testing postsymptom onset, disease severity, and patient immunostatus among other factors. As a result, over the past year, a steady influx of independent evaluations of these high-throughput assays have been published, although it is important to recognize that these studies are quite heterogeneous, varying dramatically in the types of sample sets used for accuracy analysis, including differences associated with time to sample collection relative to symptom onset, patient disease severity and age distribution, the reference method, and so on. Although this somewhat limits the ability to do direct cross-study comparisons, a high-level summary of the reported performance characteristics of commonly evaluated high-throughput assays is presented in the following section.

SARS-CoV-2 Serologic Assay Specificity

SARS-CoV-2 is the third coronavirus in the last 20 years to have spilled over from an animal reservoir to cause human disease, following SARS-CoV in 2002 and Middle East respiratory syndrome coronavirus (MERS-CoV) in 2012. Although SARS-CoV and MERS-CoV are no longer widely circulating, 4 endemic CoVs continue to cause typically mild, upper respiratory tract infections worldwide, including HKU1, OC43, 229E, and NL63. Therefore, a primary concern among both manufacturers and laboratorians considering implementing SARS-CoV-2 serologic tests was what level of specificity could such assays achieve given that greater than 65% of children and greater than 90% of adults older than 50 years are seropositive for antibodies to at least one of the commonly circulating CoVs.[21,22] At the amino acid level, the endemic CoVs share 28.4% to 34.6%, 21% to 31.2%, and 33.1% to 42.3% identity with the SARS-CoV-2 NC, S1 and S2 proteins, respectively, indicating that antibody cross-reactivity is possible among these viruses.[23,24]

Several approaches have been taken to assess assay specificity, including evaluation of samples collected before the pandemic, and in samples collected from patients with confirmed, alternative CoV or other respiratory pathogen infections. Using the Abbott SARS-CoV-2 IgG chemiluminescent microparticle immunoassay (CMIA; NC-based assay), Brecher and colleagues showed 100% specificity of this method among 20 sera collected from patients at least 30 days from polymerase chain reaction–confirmed infection with one of the 4 endemic CoVs.[25] Subsequent, larger studies using cross-reactivity and prepandemic healthy donor panels have likewise documented somewhat more variable, although still high, specificity levels for the Abbot IgG CMIA (97.5%–100%). Interestingly, using prepandemic samples collected from patients in Nigeria, a recent study showed a 6.1% false positivity rate for the Abbott IgG CMIA among 212 samples with high levels of antimalaria antibodies.[26] This unexpected cross-reactivity, which can be substantially minimized using urea treatment, has not yet been replicated with other assays. The other frequently used anti-NC based assay is the Roche total antibody anti-NC electro-chemiluminescence immunoassay (ECLIA), for which studies have consistently reported exceedingly high specificity ranges greater than 99% (**Table 2**).[10,27–29] Among the NC-based ELISAs, the Bio-Rad Platelia assay has been most frequently evaluated, with slightly lower overall specificity reported, ranging from 95% to 100% using similar panels (see **Table 2**).[28,29]

Most of the high-throughput SARS-CoV-2 serologic assays are based on recombinant spike protein components, either S1 or RBD, or a combination. The reported specificity range for CIA-based anti-S assays is similarly high as that observed for NC-based methods, typically greater than 99% (see **Table 2**). Two frequently evaluated S-based assays for which lower specificities have more been reported include the DiaSorin S1/S2 IgG CIA and the Euroimmun S1 IgG ELISA.[10,27–32] Among the studies evaluating the DiaSorin IgG CIA, Turbett and colleagues demonstrated statistically significant ($P<.005$) lower specificity of this assay in more than 1200 prepandemic samples, as compared with the Abbott IgG CIA and the Roche Total antibody ECLIA (ie, 97.8% vs 99.3% and 99.7%, respectively).[31] Jääskeläinen and colleagues report the lowest specificity for both the DiaSorin IgG CIA and the Euroimmun IgG ELISA at 91.4% and 87.7%, respectively.[10] Although these data are based on a small cross-reactivity panel set (N = 81 samples), this study is among the few to attempt to identify the potential causes of cross-reactivity, although no consistent cause was determined for these 2 assays.

Implementing highly specific SARS-CoV-2 serologic assays is essential in order to maximize the positive predictive value of results. Although this concept remains important today, this was essential early during the pandemic when prevalence of SARS-CoV-2 in the community was low—low prevalence, coupled with lower assay specificity characteristics, is associated with low positive predictive values, leading to higher rates of false-positive results.[19] Minimum serologic assay specificity thresholds have been recommended by the Centers of Disease Control and Prevention and FDA (ie, $\geq$99.5%) and the WHO (ie, $\geq$97%).[5,20,33]

SARS-CoV-2 Serologic Assay Sensitivity

The sensitivity of any serologic assay for detection of antibodies to an infectious pathogen is affected by several factors, including the limit of detection of the assay itself for

Table 2
Summary of peer-reviewed performance characteristics of select high-throughput serologic assays for SARS-CoV-2

Manufacturer/ Method	Antibody Targeted/ SARS-CoV-2 Antigen	Reported % Sensitivity		Reported % Specificity Prepandemic Samples and/ or Other Infections	Reference
		≤14 d PSO	15–150 d PSO		
Abbott/CMIA[a]	IgG/NC	40.5%–81.8%	64%–100%	97.5%–100%	10,27–32,43,46–50
Bio-Rad/ELISA	Total Ab/NC	67.8%–83%	86.7%–100%	95%–100%	28,29,46,50
Beckman/CIA	IgG/RBD	29.7%–56%	58.3%–86.7%	99.8%–100%	28,29,43
DiaSorin/CIA	IgG/S1:S2	38.5%–70.8%	54.2%–90.9%	91.4%–100%	9,10,28–31,46,50,51
EUROIMMUN/ELISA	IgG/S1	27.5%–48%	73%–100%	87.7%–100%	10,27–30,32,46,52
Ortho Clinical/CIA	IgG/S1	38.5%–84.8%	79.3%–97.0%	98%–100%	9,27,29,30,48
Ortho Clinical/CIA	Total Ab/S1	61.4%–100%	90%–100%	99%–100%	9,29,30,48
Siemens/CIA	Total Ab/RBD	32.4%–73.3%	84%–97%	99%–99.5%	29,30,43,50
Roche/ECLIA[a]	Total Ab/NC	37.8%–72.3%	73%–100%	99.1%–100%	9,28–30,32,43,46–53
Roche/ECLIA	Total Ab/RBD	61.5%–90.9%	83.3%–100%	100%	9,48,53

Abbreviations: CIA, chemiluminescent immunoassay; CMIA, chemiluminescent microparticle immunoassay; ELISA, enzyme-linked immunosorbent assay; NC, nucleocapsid; PSO, postsymptom onset; RBD, receptor binding domain; S, spike glycoprotein; S1, spike glycoprotein subunit 1; S2, spike glycoprotein subunit 2.
[a] Qualitative assay.

the target analyte, the ability of the patient to produce antibodies, and the timing of patient sampling following infection. Focusing on the latter, the temporal evolution of a humoral immune response to SARS-CoV-2 follows that of most other viral pathogens and has been discussed in detail elsewhere.[24] Using various serologic methods (most without FDA EUA), which were based on a variety of SARS-CoV-2 target antigens to detect either IgM- or IgG-specific antibodies, the growing body of evidence indicates that most of the infected individuals will develop a humoral immune response to SARS-CoV-2 within 7 to 14 days of symptom onset, with detectable IgM and IgG class antibodies evolving concurrently or closely following one another.[18,19,24] Although the duration of antibody positivity continues to be assessed, as most other viral infections, anti-SARS-CoV-2 IgM antibodies begin to decline 20 to 30 days following symptom onset. With respect to durability of anti-SARS-CoV-2 IgG antibodies, there have been conflicting reports, with some studies showing rapid decline in titers 3 to 4 months postsymptom onset, whereas others report persistent detection for 6 months or longer.[34–37] Although some of this discrepancy is likely due to variability in the assays themselves, it is increasingly apparent that immune responses are also affected by disease severity, immunocompetence, age, and sex, among other factors.[38,39]

The sensitivity of high-throughput SARS-CoV-2 serologic assays has been independently assessed for multiple different platforms, and an overarching summary, separated based on days postsymptom onset (PSO), is presented in **Table 2**. In samples from acutely symptomatic patients, collected within 14 days PSO, regardless of the SARS-CoV-2 antigen target and antibody class detected, the sensitivity of these assays is low and variable. Intraassay variability was also notable among studies evaluating the same method; this was particularly apparent in acute phase samples (eg, Abbott IgG CMIA range 42.5%–81.8%, DiaSorin IgG CIA range 38.5%–70.8%, Ortho Clinical IgG CIA range 38.5%–84.8%). As mentioned earlier, aside from method differences, assay sensitivity is also affected by the severity of disease experienced by the patient, with data showing that hospitalized patients in general develop antibodies sooner and at higher titers as compared with mildly ill or asymptomatic individuals.[36,40–42] Regardless of method, however, sensitivity increases dramatically among samples collected at least 15 days PSO, with most assays approaching 100% sensitivity at these later time points (see **Table 2**). Interestingly, the one assay that did not reach at least 90% sensitivity among samples collected 15 days or longer PSO was the Beckman IgG CIA. Although based on a low to moderate number of samples (N = 24, 30 or 176) from symptomatic patients, 3 separate studies evaluating the Beckman IgG CIA, an anti-RBD assay, reported sensitivities of 74%, 79%, and 86.7% among samples collected at later timepoints PSO[28,29,43]; this is notably discordant with the 96.8% to 100% positive percent agreement indicated by the manufacturer and as published on the FDA Website for this assay.[6] In an effort to optimize the performance characteristics of the assay, Therrien and colleagues proposed an alternative cut-off threshold for the Beckman IgG CIA, which improved sensitivity to 100% without substantially affecting specificity.[29] Although further study of the Beckman IgG CIA is warranted, this underscores the importance of independent clinical assessment of these assays in local hospitals and health care systems before assay implementation.

FUTURE OUTLOOK FOR SARS-CoV-2 SEROLOGIC TESTING

Despite initial excitement for SARS-CoV-2 serologic assays, their clinical role and utilization in the laboratory has remained minimal, as evidenced by the relatively low volume of test requests (personal observation, E. S. Theel, 2020). The reason behind this is multifold, including the lack of a well-defined correlate or surrogate of protective immunity, the inherent heterogeneity among currently available serologic assays, and as a result, the limited clinical actions that can be taken based on results from these tests. Although a positive anti-SARS-CoV-2 result indicates previous infection or vaccination (depending on the assay used), what remains undefined is the minimal antibody "threshold" associated with long-term protective immunity, as exists for other vaccine preventable diseases.[17,44] It is clear that both natural infection and vaccination are associated with protection for at least 6 to 9 months; however, it is also evident, as discussed earlier, that antibody titers can be quite variable among individuals, in both their levels and persistence.[15,16,34,45] Once such a threshold is established and the availability of SARS-CoV-2 vaccines stabilizes, results from SARS-CoV-2 serologic tests may provide more value—for example, they may be used to identify individuals who may benefit from revaccination.

Alongside the identification of a "minimum" antibody threshold associated with protective immunity, there will be a need to standardize SARS-CoV-2 serologic assays. Most of the current assays are qualitative; however, increasingly, manufacturers are developing semiquantitative assays, which provide a quantitative value typically in AU/mL. Although these values provide a general sense of antibody "levels", these semiquantitative assays are not standardized (as of the writing of the article) to the WHO SARS-CoV-2 immunoglobulin reference and therefore are not standardized to each other.[8] Such standardization will be necessary in the future to increase the clinical value of SARS-CoV-2 serologic test results.

SUMMARY

Serologic assays for SARS-CoV-2 emerged exceedingly rapidly in the early days of the pandemic, from both established and new *in vitro* diagnostic manufacturers. The ability to perform independent clinical evaluations of these assays was initially challenging due to limited reagent availability, lack of sufficient patient samples, and an unclear understanding of both how to verify assays with FDA EUA and how the humoral immune response to SARS-CoV-2 evolves, ultimately leading to the absence of an ideal reference standard for assay/result comparison. Over the past 6 months, however, more detailed, independently performed studies have been published outlining the performance characteristics of the commonly implemented high-throughput SARS-CoV-2 serologic assays (see **Table 2**). As this review has summarized, the reported specificity for most of these assays is exceedingly high, greater than 98% among both prepandemic and cross-reactivity panels. As with most other anti-viral serologic assays, sensitivity is poor to low during the first week PSO for most of the patients, increasing dramatically among samples collected at least 14 days after disease onset. Although most high-throughput assays approached 100% sensitivity at these later time points, some assays did not (eg, Beckman IgG CIA, DiaSorin IgG CIA), further underscoring the importance of clinical validation of assays before implementation (see **Table 2**). The role of serologic testing for SARS-CoV-2 in the future remains difficult to predict. The clinical utility of these assays will likely remain limited, given that most individuals will have been naturally infected or vaccinated. However, there may be a future role of SARS-CoV-2 serologic assays comparable with what is currently the case for other vaccine preventable diseases. Once a correlate of immunity is identified, testing individuals to determine whether a vaccine booster is necessary, especially if individuals are unable to provide documentation of vaccination, or to confirm immunity as is done for other vaccine-preventable diseases before arriving on campus or starting a job in health care may become a key role for these assays. In this case, high-throughput, specific SARS-CoV-2 serologic tests, primarily targeting detection of spike protein components, will be key to fill this need.

CLINICS CARE POINTS

- Despite the circulation of 4 endemic coronaviruses, most of the commonly implemented high-throughput SARS-CoV-2 serologic assays have exceedingly high specificity, minimizing the risk of false-positive results.
- The sensitivity of high-throughput SARS-CoV-2 serologic assays is best after at least 14 days postsymptom onset.
- The clinical utility of these assays is currently minimal, as they cannot be used to routinely establish a diagnosis of active COVID-19.
- Future optimization of current and new SARS-CoV-2 serologic tests should focus on standardizing these assays to an international reference standard and on the identification of a correlate of immunity against reinfection and/or disease manifestation.

DISCLOSURE

The author has participated on advisory boards for Roche Diagnostics and Accelerate Diagnostics and is on the scientific advisory board for Serimmun Inc.

REFERENCES

1. M G. Antibody testing can help open the economy and get us working again. The Hill. Available at: https://thehill.com/opinion/healthcare/491423-antibody-testing-can-help-open-the-economy-and-get-us-working-again2020. Accessed April 10, 2021.
2. Flaherty A, Abdelmalek M, L B. Could a simple blood test for COVID-19 anti-bodies help reopoen the economy? ABCNews. 2020. Available at: https://abcnewsgocom/Politics/simple-blood-test-covid-19-antibodies-reopen-economy/story?id=70024837. Accessed April 10, 2021.
3. Theel ES, Slev P, Wheeler S, et al. The role of antibody testing for SARS-CoV-2: is there one? J Clin Microbiol 2020;58(8). e00797-20.
4. Hanson KE, Caliendo AMAA, Englund JA, et al. Infectious diseases Society of America guidelines on the diagnosis of COVID-19: serologic testing. Infectious diseases Society of America 2020; version 1.0.0. Available at: https://www.idsociety.org/practice-guideline/covid-19-guideline-serology/. Accessed April 20, 2021.
5. CDC. Interim Guidelines for COVID-19 antibody testing in clinical and public health settings. Centers for Disease Control and Prevention; 2021. Available at: https://www.cdc.gov/coronavirus/2019-ncov/lab/resources/antibody-tests-guidelines.html#. Accessed April 20, 2021.
6. FDA. In vitro diagnostics EUA. Available at: https://www.fda.gov/medical-devices/coronavirus-disease-2019-covid-19-emergency-use-authorizations-medical-devices/in-vitro-diagnostics-euas. Accessed April 20, 2021. In: Administration UFaD, ed2021.
7. FDA. Removal lists of tests that should no longer be used and/or distributed for COVID-19: FAQs on testing for SARS-CoV-2. Available at: https://www.fda.gov/

medical-devices/coronavirus-covid-19-and-medical-devices/removal-lists-tests-should-no-longer-be-used-andor-distributed-covid-19-faqs-testing-sars-cov-2. Accessed April 20, 2021.

8. Mattiuzzo G, Bently EM, Hassall M, et al. Establishment of the WHO international standard and reference panel for anti-SARS-CoV-2 antibody. In: WHO, editor. WHO. Geneva (Switzerland): WHO; 2020. p. 1–60.

9. Favresse J, Eucher C, Elsen M, et al. Persistence of anti-SARS-CoV-2 antibodies depends on the analytical kit: a report for up to 10 Months after infection. Microorganisms 2021;9(3):556.

10. Jaaskelainen AJ, Kuivanen S, Kekalainen E, et al. Performance of six SARS-CoV-2 immunoassays in comparison with microneutralisation. J Clin Virol 2020;129: 104512.

11. Ou X, Liu Y, Lei X, et al. Characterization of spike glycoprotein of SARS-CoV-2 on virus entry and its immune cross-reactivity with SARS-CoV. Nat Commun 2020; 11(1):1620.

12. Zeng W, Liu G, Ma H, et al. Biochemical characterization of SARS-CoV-2 nucleocapsid protein. Biochem Biophys Res Commun 2020;527(3):618–23.

13. Krammer F. SARS-CoV-2 vaccines in development. Nature 2020;586(7830): 516–27.

14. Marot S, Malet I, Leducq V, et al. Rapid decline of neutralizing antibodies against SARS-CoV-2 among infected healthcare workers. Nat Commun 2021;12(1):844.

15. Jackson LA, Anderson EJ, Rouphael NG, et al. An mRNA vaccine against SARS-CoV-2 - preliminary report. N Engl J Med 2020;383(20):1920–31.

16. Polack FP, Thomas SJ, Kitchin N, et al. Safety and efficacy of the BNT162b2 mRNA Covid-19 vaccine. N Engl J Med 2020;383(27):2603–15.

17. Amanna IJ, Messaoudi I, Slifka MK. Protective immunity following vaccination: how is it defined? Hum Vaccin 2008;4(4):316–9.

18. Zhang YV, Wiencek J, Meng QH, et al. AACC practical recommendations for implementing and interpreting SARS-CoV-2 EUA and LDT serologic testing in clinical laboratories. Clin Chem 2021;67(9):1188–200.

19. Theel ES, Couturier MR, Filkins L, et al. Application, verification, and implementation of SARS-CoV-2 serologic assays with emergency use authorization. J Clin Microbiol 2020;59(1). e02148-20.

20. FDA. EUA authorized Serology test performance. 2020. Available at: https://www.fda.gov/medical-devices/coronavirus-disease-2019-covid-19-emergency-use-authorizations-medical-devices/eua-authorized-serology-test-performance. Accessed April 20, 2021.

21. Gorse GJ, Patel GB, Vitale JN, et al. Prevalence of antibodies to four human coronaviruses is lower in nasal secretions than in serum. Clin Vaccin Immunol 2010; 17(12):1875–80.

22. Principi N, Bosis S, Esposito S. Effects of coronavirus infections in children. Emerg Infect Dis 2010;16(2):183–8.

23. Okba NMA, Muller MA, Li W, et al. Severe acute respiratory syndrome coronavirus 2-specific antibody responses in coronavirus disease patients. Emerg Infect Dis 2020;26(7):1478–88.

24. Galipeau Y, Greig M, Liu G, et al. Humoral responses and serological assays in SARS-CoV-2 infections. Front Immunol 2020;11:610688.

25. Brecher SM, Dryjowicz-Burek J, Yu H, et al. Patients with Common Cold coronaviruses tested negative for IgG antibody to SARS-CoV-2. J Clin Microbiol 2020; 58(8). e01029-20.

26. Steinhardt LC, Ige F, Iriemenam NC, et al. Cross-reactivity of two SARS-CoV-2 serological assays in a malaria-endemic setting. J Clin Microbiol 2021;59(7): e0051421.
27. Theel ES, Harring J, Hilgart H, et al. Performance characteristics of four high-throughput immunoassays for detection of IgG antibodies against SARS-CoV-2. J Clin Microbiol 2020;58(8). e01243-20.
28. Plaga A, Wei R, Olson E, et al. Evaluation of the clinical performance of seven serological assays for SARS-CoV-2 for use in clinical laboratories. J Appl Lab Med 2021;6(4):998–1004.
29. Therrien C, Serhir B, Belanger-Collard M, et al. Multicenter evaluation of the clinical performance and the neutralizing antibody activity prediction properties of 10 high-throughput serological assays used in clinical laboratories. J Clin Microbiol 2021;59(3). e02511-20.
30. Harritshoj LH, Gybel-Brask M, Afzal S, et al. Comparison of sixteen serological SARS-CoV-2 immunoassays in sixteen clinical laboratories. J Clin Microbiol 2021;59(5). e02596-20.
31. Turbett SE, Anahtar M, Dighe AS, et al. Evaluation of three commercial SARS-CoV-2 serologic assays and their performance in two-test algorithms. J Clin Microbiol 2021;59(1). e01892-20.
32. Patel EU, Bloch EM, Clarke W, et al. Comparative performance of five commercially available serologic assays to detect antibodies to SARS-CoV-2 and identify individuals with high neutralizing titers. J Clin Microbiol 2021;59(2). e02257-20.
33. WHO. Target product profiles for the priority diagnostics to support the COVID-19 pandemic v.1.0. Geneva (Switzerland): WHO; 2020.
34. Dan JM, Mateus J, Kato Y, et al. Immunological memory to SARS-CoV-2 assessed for up to 8 months after infection. Science 2021;371(6529):eabf4063.
35. Gudbjartsson DF, Norddahl GL, Melsted P, et al. Humoral immune response to SARS-CoV-2 in Iceland. N Engl J Med 2020;383(18):1724–34.
36. Seow J, Graham C, Merrick B, et al. Longitudinal observation and decline of neutralizing antibody responses in the three months following SARS-CoV-2 infection in humans. Nat Microbiol 2020;5(12):1598–607.
37. Wajnberg A, Amanat F, Firpo A, et al. Robust neutralizing antibodies to SARS-CoV-2 infection persist for months. Science 2020;370(6521):1227–30.
38. Brodin P. Immune determinants of COVID-19 disease presentation and severity. Nat Med 2021;27(1):28–33.
39. Chen X, Pan Z, Yue S, et al. Disease severity dictates SARS-CoV-2-specific neutralizing antibody responses in COVID-19. Signal Transduct Target Ther 2020;5(1):180.
40. Wang Y, Zhang L, Sang L, et al. Kinetics of viral load and antibody response in relation to COVID-19 severity. J Clin Invest 2020;130(10):5235–44.
41. Wellinghausen N, Plonne D, Voss M, et al. SARS-CoV-2-IgG response is different in COVID-19 outpatients and asymptomatic contact persons. J Clin Virol 2020; 130:104542.
42. Long QX, Tang XJ, Shi QL, et al. Clinical and immunological assessment of asymptomatic SARS-CoV-2 infections. Nat Med 2020;26(8):1200–4.
43. Tan SS, Saw S, Chew KL, et al. Head-to-head evaluation on diagnostic accuracies of six SARS-CoV-2 serological assays. Pathology 2020;52(7):770–7.
44. Plotkin SA. Vaccines: correlates of vaccine-induced immunity. Clin Infect Dis 2008;47(3):401–9.
45. Lumley SF, O'Donnell D, Stoesser NE, et al. Antibody Status and incidence of SARS-CoV-2 infection in Health Care workers. N Engl J Med 2021;384(6):533–40.

46. Charlton CL, Kanji JN, Johal K, et al. Evaluation of six commercial mid- to high-volume Antibody and six point-of-Care lateral flow assays for detection of SARS-CoV-2 antibodies. J Clin Microbiol 2020;58(10). e01361-20.
47. Harley K, Gunsolus IL. Comparison of the clinical performances of the Abbott alinity IgG, Abbott architect IgM, and Roche elecsys total SARS-CoV-2 antibody assays. J Clin Microbiol 2020;59(1). e02104-20.
48. Kubota K, Kitagawa Y, Matsuoka M, et al. Clinical evaluation of the antibody response in patients with COVID-19 using automated high-throughput immuno-assays. Diagn Microbiol Infect Dis 2021;100(3):115370.
49. Parai D, Dash GC, Choudhary HR, et al. Diagnostic accuracy comparison of three fully automated chemiluminescent immunoassay platforms for the detection of SARS-CoV-2 antibodies. J Virol Methods 2021;292:114121.
50. Trabaud MA, Icard V, Milon MP, et al. Comparison of eight commercial, high-throughput, automated or ELISA assays detecting SARS-CoV-2 IgG or total anti-body. J Clin Virol 2020;132:104613.
51. Chiereghin A, Zagari RM, Galli S, et al. Recent advances in the evaluation of sero-logical assays for the diagnosis of SARS-CoV-2 infection and COVID-19. Front Public Health 2020;8:620222.
52. Heffernan E, Kennedy L, Hannan M, et al. EXPRESS: performance characteristics of five SARS-CoV-2 serological assays: clinical utility in healthcare workers. Ann Clin Biochem 2021. 45632211012728.
53. Poljak M, Ostrbenk Valencak A, Stamol T, et al. Head-to-head comparison of two rapid high-throughput automated electrochemiluminescence immunoassays tar-geting total antibodies to the SARS-CoV-2 nucleoprotein and spike protein recep-tor binding domain. J Clin Virol 2021;137:104784.

Performance Evaluation of Lateral Flow Assays for Coronavirus Disease-19 Serology

Lucy Ochola, PhD[a], Paul Ogongo, PhD[a,b], Samuel Mungai, MS[c],
Jesse Gitaka, MB ChB, PhD[c], Sara Suliman, MPH, PhD[b,d],*

KEYWORDS

- COVID-19 • SARS-CoV-2 • LFAs • Diagnostics • Serology

KEY POINTS

- Lateral flow assays (LFAs) are affordable and easy-to-use serologic assays for SARS-CoV-2.
- LFAs are amenable for home testing and community seroprevalence monitoring efforts.
- Evaluation of LFAs includes both laboratory assessment of performance characteristics and fitness for implementation.
- The utility of LFAs should adapt to vaccine rollouts and emergence of new SARS-CoV-2 variant strains.

INTRODUCTION

The coronavirus disease of 2019 (COVID-19), caused by infection with the severe acute respiratory syndrome coronavirus-2 (SARS-CoV-2) has undoubtedly been the most disruptive pandemic of the last century.[1] Despite global advances in testing, the true burden of COVID-19 in most countries still remains unclear and is continuously evolving.[2] Reports of prevalence rates thus far have relied on positive SARS-CoV-2 diagnosis using gold standard molecular diagnostics and rapid antigen tests.[3] On the other hand, seroprevalence studies estimate the rates of prior exposure to the virus in each population by gauging the proportion of individuals with antibodies against the virus.[4,5] These estimates of the true extent of herd immunity in different

[a] Department of Tropical and Infectious Diseases, Institute of Primate Research, National Museums of Kenya, PO Box 24481, Nairobi 00502, Kenya; [b] Division of Experimental Medicine, Department of Medicine, University of California, San Francisco, San Francisco, CA 94143, USA; [c] Directorate of Research and Innovation, Mount Kenya University, PO Box 342-01000, Thika, Kenya; [d] Division of Rheumatology, Inflammation and Immunity, Brigham and Women's Hospital, Boston, MA 02115, USA
* Corresponding author. UCSF at Zuckerberg San Francisco General Hospital, 1001 Potrero Avenue, Building 3, Room 509A, Box 1234, San Francisco, CA 94110.
E-mail address: sara.suliman@ucsf.edu

Clin Lab Med 42 (2022) 31–56
https://doi.org/10.1016/j.cll.2021.10.005
0272-2712/22/© 2021 Elsevier Inc. All rights reserved.

labmed.theclinics.com

communities[6,7] could inform public health action and unveil disparities in the susceptibilities of diverse communities to infection with SARS-CoV-2.[8,9] As several vaccines are administered globally,[10] monitoring longevity of immune responses induced by vaccination or natural infection with SARS-CoV-2 should inform public health measures to prioritize high-risk populations, such as informal settlements with lower socioeconomic statuses,[11] for vaccinations or to implement containment measures, such as lockdowns and travel restrictions. Serologic lateral flow assays (LFAs) provide an affordable and scalable solution to rapidly monitor seroprevalence and attainment of herd immunity.[12,13]

Here, we review the global context and use cases in which serologic tests are deployed, with a specific focus on LFAs. We review considerations for designing studies to evaluate LFAs, particularly in the context of COVID-19 vaccinations and emerging SARS-CoV-2 variants and provide guidance for implementation of LFAs for both home use and population surveillance.

SARS-CoV-2 Diagnostics

To date, diagnosis has played an important role in monitoring and managing SARS-CoV-2 infections.[14] COVID-19 tests can be broadly classified into molecular diagnostics, antigen-detection tests (rapid tests), and serologic diagnostics, which detect anti-SARS-CoV-2 antibodies.[3,15] Molecular and antigen tests detect active viral infections, whereas serologic tests indicate prior exposure to the virus by measuring SARS-CoV-2-specific antibodies.[16,17] Gold-standard point-of-care molecular tests currently rely on the detection of ribonucleic acid (RNA) from SARS-CoV-2 by reverse transcriptase-quantitative polymerase chain reactions (RT-qPCR).[18] Rapid antigen tests detect viral antigens, and offer an attractive option for affordable and scalable diagnostics, especially for mass community surveillance.[19–21] However, both molecular and rapid antigen tests only detect active infections, and do not assess prior exposure to SARS-CoV-2, the extent of transmission that had already occurred in a population, or immune status and durability of antibody responses.[22] Serologic tests can be useful epidemiologic tools for monitoring the infection prevalence and herd immunity in diverse populations.[4] As LFAs are cheap and scalable, they are the most amenable form of serologic assays to fulfill these individual and epidemiologic needs.[4]

Need for Validated Serologic Tests for Coronavirus Disease of 2019

Since the beginning of the pandemic, diagnostic tests and serologic assays have flooded the market. Test developers took advantage of the emergency use authorization (EUA) process by the Food and Drug Administration (FDA) locally,[23] and regulatory bodies internationally, including the European Commission, Ministry of Health in Canada, Medicines and Healthcare products Regulatory Agency (MHRA) in the United Kingdom, and the World Health Organization (WHO), to release their products to the market before completing detailed evaluations.[24] Many serologic tests obtained EUA by the FDA,[23] or equivalent regulatory approvals, for example, interim order (IO) authorizations or Conformité Européenne (CE) marks, with evaluations that were often based on samples from a small number of patients, which were not always representative of the entire susceptible population (e.g., symptomatic patients only).[25] Therefore, these evaluations limited the reliability and generalizability of tests to estimate the true extent of SARS-CoV-2 transmission in diverse community settings. Hence, standardized protocols for rigorous evaluations of these tests by manufacturer-independent third parties became crucial to determine their accuracy and usability in an unbiased way.[26] Importantly, the increased reliance on antibody tests as "immunity passports" demands their careful evaluation, as well as community education on the interpretation of the test results, to prevent premature assumptions of immunity against SARS-CoV-2.[27–29]

World Health Organization Guidance on Serologic Testing

Since mid-2020, the WHO has advocated for countrywide serosurveys to determine the extent of SARS-CoV-2 spread globally.[30] To guide this process, the WHO developed an interim guidance policy document stating that serologic assays would be crucial to support serosurveillance efforts aimed at estimating transmission to inform public health responses.[31] However, in this document,[30] the WHO cautioned against using serologic assays to determine antibody titers as surrogates for protective immunity, or as tools for contact tracing or diagnosis of active infections.[30,31]

To support country-wide serosurveillance efforts, the WHO partnered with the Centers for Disease Control (CDC), the Foundation for Innovative New Diagnostics (FINDdx), African Society for Laboratory Medicine (ASLM), and others, to evaluate and roll out COVID-19 diagnostics.[32] As a result, FIND created a centralized repository of available SARS-CoV-2 serologic assays,[32] which measures both performance accuracy and feasibility for scale-up in low and middle-income countries. This effort resulted in standardized protocols to evaluate the accuracy and suitability of serologic assays to achieve the following: triaging suspected patients with COVID-19, assessing recovery of convalescent patients with COVID-19, and implementation of these assays in broader seroprevalence initiatives to inform public health actions, such as prioritizing regions of high transmission, for COVID-19 vaccination. Easy-to-use serologic assays, such as LFAs, which are also affordable and scalable, will be key to decentralizing access to these tests.[33]

Seroprevalence of Severe Acute Respiratory Syndrome Coronavirus 2 Globally

Several reports conducted in different populations with varied demographics showed a wide range of seroprevalence estimates of antibodies against SARS-CoV-2, as highlighted herein.[5] In Wuhan, China, a study on samples from 18,712 asymptomatic participants collected between January and February 2020 found a seroprevalence of 3%-8% for IgG titers,[34] whereas another study in the same area from March to April 2020 described rates of 0.3% in 9442 community resident men.[35] In the United States, one study had 4675 outpatients,[36] another 177,919 community samples,[37] and in the United Kingdom, 365,000 community samples yielded rates that varied from 0% to 20%.[38] In a Spanish teaching hospital in Madrid, seroprevalence estimates ranged from 25% to 33% among 2919 health care workers.[39] In a slum in India, the seroprevalence was as high as 57.9% in 470 individuals.[13] In Pakistan, the estimates in Karachi ranged from 8.7% to 15.1% for 3005 community samples.[40]

In sub-Saharan Africa (SSA), most economies adopted systematic lockdowns, social distancing, and donning of masks to reduce transmission.[41,42] As a result, SSA countries saw overall lower rates of severe disease in the early stages of the pandemic.[43–45] However, following the economic pressure to reopen and relaxation of social distancing measures, infection rates have risen, with seroprevalence estimates in Kenya between 5% for 3174 blood donor samples[46] and 50% for 196 antenatal clinical samples,[47] 12.3% among 500 asymptomatic health care workers in Malawi,[48] 3% of 99 asymptomatic individuals sampled in Ethiopia,[49] 45% in 133 health care workers in Nigeria,[50] Guinea Bissau 18% in 140 health care workers,[51] and 38.5% among 2214 individuals in households in South Sudan.[52] However, in most cases, these estimates are based on studies of target groups, such as health care workers, truck drivers, and small populations of less than 3,000 individuals.[5,53] Therefore, the number of participants in SARS-CoV-2 serosurveys in low- and middle-income countries has been generally lower than those of wealthier counterparts. The true extent of COVID-19 spread, particularly in rural settings with little active case finding and surveillance remains undetermined, especially whereby social distancing measures are more difficult to enforce.[54] These seroprevalence studies collectively demonstrate that SARS-CoV-2 spread, estimated by molecular test positivity rates, severely underestimate true transmission rates.[5,55] Therefore, there is a need for more systematic sampling to determine the evolving seroprevalence of COVID-19 across various communities.

Types of Serologic Tests for Severe Acute Respiratory Syndrome Coronavirus 2

Serologic tests that detect antibodies against SARS-CoV-2 include enzyme-linked immunosorbent assays (ELISAs), chemiluminescence assays, and LFAs.[56–59] ELISAs are plate-based assays to detect an analyte, such as an antibody against a SARS-CoV-2 antigen. Several commercial and noncommercial tests have been developed to measure antibodies to SARS-CoV-2, which include both ELISA[60] and chemiluminescence immunoassays.[61] These assays generally target antibodies against the receptor-binding domain (RBD), spike (S), or nucleocapsid (N) proteins.[60,61] The commercially developed ELISA EUROIMMUN assay detects IgA/IgG antibodies that bind to spike antigens.[62–64] This ELISA has been evaluated using 103 clinical samples, whereby they observed a sensitivity of 21.6% within a week of symptoms onset, 55.1% on the second week and 89.5% after 2 weeks for IgG, with an overall specificity of 96.1%. Similar results were obtained for NovaLisa ELISA kit at 2-weeks post-infection for IgG (sensitivity: 94.9%, specificity: 96.2%), IgM (sensitivity: 89.7%, specificity: 98.7%), and IgA (sensitivity: 48.7%, specificity: 98.7%) in 287 patients. The Platelia ELISA kit yielded 97.4% and 94.9% sensitivity and specificity, respectively[65], using the same 287 patient samples. Several in-house noncommercial ELISAs have also been developed. A recent study evaluated inactivated SARS-CoV-2 virus antigen by ELISA using 513 clinical samples at 2-weeks postinfection and found that it demonstrated 92.3% sensitivity and 97.9% specificity.[66] An alternative indirect ELISA method used S protein to measure IgG to SARS-CoV-2 in 418 healthy persons, patients with COVID-19 and health care workers, yielding 100% sensitivity and 98.4% specificity, with no cross-reactivity to other human coronaviruses.[67] In another study, 30 inpatients with SARS-CoV-2-positive were subdivided into severe and mild, based on whether they needed intensive care or not, respectively, and a total of 151 samples were collected.[68] In these samples, evaluation of IgG titers of RBD, S, and N proteins showed that antibodies against RBD and N proteins more accurately reflected disease status, and were higher in samples from inpatients with severe than mild COVID-19.[68] For chemiluminescent assays, the sensitivity was 96% in 1338 clinical samples collected at a median of 47 days.[69] Although ELISAs and chemiluminescent assays can quantify antibodies, they remain primarily a research tool, particularly in resource-limited areas, since they require expensive equipment, trained personnel, and central laboratories that preclude their use in decentralized community testing programs.

Serologic LFAs are best suited as point-of-care tests for assessing prior exposure to SARS-CoV-2.[4,70] LFAs were thus developed as tools to detect SARS-CoV-2-specific antibodies in patient sera, plasma, or whole blood. Earlier in the pandemic, serologic LFAs were proposed as alternatives to the expensive and time-intensive RT-qPCR, to complement COVID-19 diagnosis.[71,72] However, molecular and rapid antigen tests remain the gold standard for diagnosing active infection. LFAs are simple devices that usually show a qualitative band to indicate the presence of antibodies targeting different SARS-CoV-2 antigens, and usually a second control band to indicate the validity of the test. SARS-CoV-2 serologic LFAs are effective in detecting antibodies between 15 and 30 days after the onset of disease.[33,58,73,74] However, data on the sensitivity of the LFAs more than 30-days postinfection are limited. There are currently more than 448 tests available or in development (SARS-CoV-2 diagnostic pipeline - FIND (finddx.org)). The FINDdx repository continues to be updated with new SARS-CoV-2 serologic tests and their performance characteristics, as evaluated by multiple partner institutions,[32] (**Fig. 1**, **Table 1**). The performance of these assays relies on the ability of SARS-CoV-2-infected individuals to mount antibodies against the virus as described later in discussion.

Induction of Antibodies Against Severe Acute Respiratory Syndrome Coronavirus 2

Innate and adaptive immunity play an important role in controlling SARS-CoV-2 infection.[75] Adaptive immunity creates durable memory responses to reinfection with SARS-CoV-2, through T cell-mediated cellular immunity,[75–77] and B cell-mediated humoral immunity.[78,79] B cells differentiate into plasma cells, which produce antibodies that target viral antigens. Binding of antibodies to the virus can neutralize it and block its replication in host cells, which forms the basis for proposed antibody therapeutics against SARS-CoV-2.[80,81] Antibodies against SARS-CoV-2 include multiple isotypes[82]: immunoglobulin-M (IgM), IgG, IgA, which start to appear in patients with COVID-19 around 7 to 14 days post-infection and persist for weeks after virus clearance.[83] The most detected antibodies recognize either the internal N protein or the highly immunogenic external S protein.[84] The RBD is the component of the spike

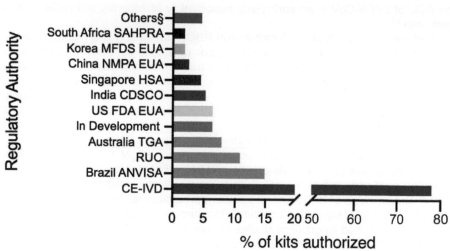

Fig. 1. Regulatory Authorizations for COVID-19 Serology LFAs: The percentage of serology lateral flow kits (x-axis) that have been approved by different regulatory bodies across the world (y-axis). Others§: combination of regulatory authorities that have approved less than 1% of the kits (n = 269), including the Philippines FDA and Korea Export (0.7% each), CO-FEPRIS (Comisión Federal para la Protección contra Riesgos Sanitarios; Mexico), In Vitro Diagnostics class D (IVD-D), Ministry of Health, Labor and Welfare-In Vitro Diagnostics (MHLW-IVD), Medicines and Healthcare Products Regulatory Agency (MHRA; UK), Medical Device Authority (MDA; Malaysia), Roszdravnadzor (RZN; Russia), Swiss Medic and Taiwan FDA (0.4% each). CE-IVD: Conformité Européene In vitro diagnostics (approval by the EU). RUO: Research Use Only. EUA: Emergency Use Authorization. Data is accessed from the Foundation for Innovative New Diagnostics (FINDdx).[32]

Table 1
COVID-19 Lateral Flow Serology Assays Reported by Foundation for Innovative New Diagnostics (FIND), accessed on 02 April 2021

Feature/Characteristic	Total: n (%)
Target antibody	269 (100%)
IgG	269 (100%)
IgM	269 (100%)
Type of sample to test	269 (100%)
Serum	269 (100%)
Plasma	269 (100%)
Whole Blood	269 (100%)
Phase of development	269 (100%)
Commercialized	250 (92.9%)
In development	19 (7.1%)
Use authorization	269 (100%)
Emergency Use Authorization	29 (10.8%)
Research Use Only	29 (10.8%)
No restricted use	211 (78.4%)

protein, which binds to the human angiotensin-converting enzyme-2 (ACE2) receptor to enter and replicate in the host cell.[85,86] Therefore, neutralizing antibodies against the RBD of SARS-CoV-2 are particularly important to block entry and replication in host cells.[87]

Given the integral role of the S protein and RBD in facilitating viral entry, these antigens form the basis of many immunoassays described to date[87,88] and inform rational COVID-19 vaccine design.[89] Recent data from immunoassays based on the SARS-CoV-2 nucleocapsid protein show high sensitivity.[33,58,90,91] However, the higher sequence homology of the SARS-CoV-2 N protein to other coronaviruses, than the S protein, could increase the possibility of cross-reactivity against N proteins from related coronaviruses.[92–94]

IgM antibodies are usually the first humoral response on SARS-CoV-2 infection.[95] Travel requirements in China have required a negative IgM test to permit travel (http://www.china-embassy.org/eng/notices/t1841416.htm). However, using IgM as an indicator of early infection is still likely to miss individuals within 5 days of exposure.[62] Serum levels of SARS-CoV-2-specific IgM antibodies decrease precipitously over time, than IgG response, as shown in longitudinal serosurveys of households in Wuhan, China,[95] and longitudinal studies of convalescent patients after discharge.[77] In contrast, SARS-CoV-2 RBD-specific IgG antibodies were durable in convalescent patients with COVID-19 and showed minimal cross-reactivity against other widely circulating coronaviruses (HKU1, 229E, OC43, NL63).[96]

Utility of Lateral Flow Assays for Coronavirus Disease of 2019 Antibody Testing

LFAs are effective point-of-care tools to detect immune responses to widely transmitted infections like SARS-CoV-2.[97,98] Serologic LFAs measure pathogen-specific antibodies in accessible biological specimens using simple platforms, whereby gold or other material-based nanoparticles are often used to label secondary antibodies.[98,99] LFAs are ideal for mass population surveillance for antibody responses, induced by either natural infection or vaccination, because they are cost-effective, portable, rapid, can be designed to measure more than one antibody isotype in the same sample, and do not require sophisticated equipment to produce results.[4,97] Furthermore, LFAs are easy-to-use and do not require specialized training for implementation.[100] Additional developments to improve their sensitivity include the use of smartphone apps to detect positive LFA results, which could enable aggregation of data in centralized databases to report disease exposure and inform public health intervention.[99,101] Therefore, LFAs are useful candidates for population serosurveillance and to monitor longevity of vaccine and SARS-CoV-2-induced antibodies to understand the real extent of herd immunity in a population.[6,102] However, before implementation of LFAs, the performance of these assays must be systematically evaluated (**Table 2**), including the impact of factors such as temperature and humidity.[25,32,103]

Band Strength and Sensitivity of Lateral Flow Assays

As LFAs are designed to be qualitative tests, an important question is whether the band strength (that is, the color intensity of the bands) should be evaluated. The interpretation of band strength can be subjective, but perhaps can be improved by incorporating smartphone apps, as conducted recently for a rapid antigen test.[104] Variation in band strength across multiple samples raises the question of whether band strength correlates with titers of antibody titers.[105] Antibody levels, determined by optical density (OD) ratios, were initially low following symptom onset, then increased over time whereby IgM, IgG, and IgA levels correlated with clinical disease severity.[106] A rapid decay of anti-SARS-CoV-2 antibodies, particularly for patients with mild symptoms implies that the band intensity could serve as a biomarker for disease severity.[107] As suboptimal antibody titers may promote pathology through antibody dependent-enhancement,[108] correlating LFA band strength with symptom severity could provide a use case for LFAs to inform clinical management. Because LFAs are best suited for population surveillance, the importance of the analytical sensitivity, also known as the limit of detection (LoD) of LFA, that is, the lowest antibody titers in each sample to give a positive LFA result, cannot be understated. High analytical sensitivity is important in cases that present late with milder symptoms and in patients suspected of COVID-19 despite a negative SARS-CoV-2 RT-qPCR test result.[90]

Use Cases of Serologic Lateral Flow Assays

LFAs have the potential of deployment outside of clinical care settings due to their affordability and ease of use.[4] The number of people infected with SARS-CoV-2 is known to be underestimated, especially in low- and middle-income countries,[47] due to the high rate of unreported and asymptomatic cases which can spread the infection within the community.[109] The availability of molecular testing and public health restrictions that follow especially for the informal labor sector and rural communities, pose real barriers to testing.[9] Thus, LFAs provide a cheap and scalable alternative to estimate the spread in diverse communities. The presence of anti-SARS-CoV-2 antibodies can identify presumably immune individuals and could thus serve as a tool to release individuals from isolation or lockdown.[103] However, it is important to note that LFAs do not quantify antibody titers or their neutralizing potential. Hence, LFAs are not ideal surrogates for herd immunity,[6,102] but are better suited for estimating SARS-CoV-2 transmission in diverse communities.

On the individual level, LFAs can complement efforts for retrospective diagnosis of presumably exposed individuals.[94] Positive LFA results can confirm exposure to a SARS-CoV-2-infected individual, and so LFAs can complement contact-tracing tools, but cannot replace molecular or antigen tests.[94] LFAs are also ideal as direct-to-

Table 2
Key considerations for LFA evaluation studies

	Issues and Questions to Address in the Evaluation
Target population	• Will the study include both symptomatic and asymptomatic individuals? • Inclusion of vulnerable and high-risk populations (e.g., immunocompromised individuals and those with comorbidities)? • Diverse ethnic and socio-economic participants • Different age groups (children and the elderly) • Implementation in occupational settings: for example, for testing healthcare workers and education staff • Inclusion of travelers (e.g., for border crossing restrictions)
Sampling scheme	• Cross-sectional schemes for direct evaluation of LFA performance characteristics (e.g., sensitivity and specificity) • Longitudinal schemes particularly of highly exposed individuals to allow the analysis of seroconversion, durability of vaccine, and infection-induced antibody responses
Type of sample	• Are samples easy to collect? (e.g., finger prick whole blood, urine, saliva)? Invasiveness? • Does the sample collection require trained personnel? • Access to storage and transport conditions to preserve the sample quality • Infection control: Does the sample expose the "collector" to SARS-CoV-2 or other pathogens? • Can the end-user collect the samples themselves?
Study case definition	Confirmed SARS-CoV-2 exposure and time between confirmed RT-qPCR test and sample collection for serology.
Study control definition	1. Historic pre-pandemic samples 2. Populations that are routinely tested: For example, healthcare workers without any documented positive test
Performance characteristics	Test sensitivity Test specificity Positive predictive values (PPV) Negative predictive values (NPV)
Prevalence in the target population	• The impact of prevalence on PPV and NPV? • Would the test overestimate or underestimate the test results?
Specificity controls	• Will the evaluation determine analytical specificity by measuring cross-reactivity against other seasonal coronaviruses: HKU1, OC43, NL63, and 229E, or coronaviruses from previous outbreaks: SARS-CoV and MERS?
Reference standard	• Will the evaluation include reference serology standards: for example, pooled samples from known positives with high, mid, and low antibody titers.
Target antigen	• What is the target antigen in the LFA? 1. Nucleocapsid 2. Spike 3. Other antigens: for example, RBD

(continued on next page)

Table 2 (continued)	
	Issues and Questions to Address in the Evaluation
Isotype of interest	• Will the test target IgM, IgG, or IgA isotypes? • What is the definition of a positive and negative test result if multiple antibody isotypes are included?
Conservation of antigen	• Is the target antigen from a conserved region of the SARS-CoV-2 genomic sequence? • How similar is the antigen to other coronaviruses to allow discrimination of SARS-CoV-2? • Is the LFA performance impacted by mutations in the SARS-CoV-2 antigens?
Variants	• What autologous SARS-CoV-2 strain was the "case" infected with? • Is the LFA intended to specifically detect SARS-CoV-2 variants?
Limit of detection	• What is the analytical sensitivity of the LFA: at which antibody concentration does the LFA lose sensitivity?
Quantitative utility	• Is the kit used for qualitative test results only? • Does the band intensity correlate with antibody titers?
Vaccination Status	• Is this LFA intended for a vaccinated population?
Use cases	• Individual vs population? • Vaccinated vs unvaccinated? • Epidemiologic understanding of seroprevalence and transmission? • Durability of responses?
Financial effectiveness	• How affordable is the test? • Will the cost allow the LFA to be subsidized by a healthcare system or individuals will cover the cost? • How does the cost impact the community uptake?
Utility of implementation	• Does the LFA fulfill a critical public health implementation need? • Is the LFA the most suitable testing modality for the use case? • Do you foresee barriers to social acceptability to implementation?
Supply chain (manufacturer)	• Can manufacturing be scaled up? • Who is funding the manufacturing? • What is the availability of consumables in the region? • Will the LFA kits require assembly in the user laboratories, or is the assembly centralized? • Are the locally available consumables compatible with the LFA?
Impact on clinical decision making	• Does the result impact clinical practice? • Is there evidence supporting the implementation of the LFA in clinical care settings?
Provider/health care system acceptance	• Are the LFA vendor and/or developer considered credible for local public health authorities?
Utility for local public health systems?	• What is the demand landscape for the LFA? • Does the LFA inform social distancing guidelines? • Can the evaluation protocol determine fitness for implementation?

(continued on next page)

Table 2 (continued)	
	Issues and Questions to Address in the Evaluation
	• Is the LFA high on the priority list for tools in the fight against the COVID-19 pandemic?
	• What are the cold chain requirements for storage and distribution?
	• Can the LFA adapt to different temperatures/climates?
Feasibility and adoption	• Is there a political will to adopt LFAs?
	• What is the available infrastructure for rolling out LFAs?
	• Are they fit for the proposed use cases?
	• What is the balance between feasibility, practicality, and actual fit that ensure the utility of adoption?
	• Will the evaluation assess adoption-uptake (decision to use the LFA and trialability (ability to attract the utilization and ease of use-for direct-to-consumer testing)[160,161]?

consumer at-home serologic tests that empower individuals to test for anti-SARS-CoV-2 antibodies.[110] The Food and Drug Administration (FDA) has already approved several LFAs, such as Cellex qSARS-CoV-2 IgG/IgM Rapid Test and others for home use.[111] Interestingly, Cellex partnered with Gauss to launch a parallel rapid SARS-CoV-2 antigen test, which was the first to be approved by the FDA for home use.[112] It is very likely that serologic LFAs will follow suit. Although home use of serologic tests can be a vital instrument in empowering users, the risk of result misinterpretation is very high,[33] and may result in premature behavioral changes that could increase the risk of SARS-CoV-2 transmission. More dangerously, ineffective immunity has the chance of exerting selection pressure to increase spontaneous mutations of SARS-CoV-2, and transmission of SARS-CoV-2 variants of conern.[7,113] A positive result is prone to be false when the prevalence of the disease is low, or if the specificity of the assay is suboptimal for reasons such as cross-reactivity with related coronaviruses.[114] Therefore, deployment of LFAs for home-use requires the inclusion of educational materials that facilitate interpretation as explained later in discussion.

Lateral Flow Assays to Distinguish Antibodies Induced by Infection or Vaccination

The identity of target SARS-CoV-2 antigens in the LFAs is critical.[22,33,57,58] Some LFA kits target the N protein,[115] others the RBD[116] and some the S protein, which is displayed all around the surface of the virus.[85] Additionally, the N-terminal domain of the N protein is highly conserved in all beta-coronaviruses and may cause false-positive results and/or fail to detect true early sensitization.[94] Several widely used SARS-CoV-2 vaccines use the S antigen, including mRNA-1273 by Moderna,[117] AZD1222 by AstraZeneca,[118] the Ad26.COV2.S[119] from Johnson and Johnson, or more specifically the RBD of BTN162b2 by Pfizer-BioNTech.[120] Therefore, in populations that receive Spike-based vaccines, LFAs targeting the N and S antigens can be used to distinguish natural SARS-CoV-2 infection only, or vaccine and infection-induced antibodies, respectively (see **Table 2**). Vaccines that are based on the complete inactivated virus, such as BBV152/COVAXIN or N antigen only will not allow this use case.[121] The variety of antigenic targets for the LFAs, as well as more complex serologic assays, allow for this application.[33,122] LFAs targeting the S protein only include COVID-19 IgM/IgG tests from: Camtech, Oranoxis, and Ozo, and N-specific LFAs include CareHealth, KHB, Phamatech, and Ray Biotech, whereas several LFAs target both and would not be suitable for this use case.[33,58] The tests overall show high sensitivity and specificity for IgG antibodies in samples collected 10 days or more following a positive SARS-CoV-2 RT-qPCR result.[33] The sensitivity was generally higher for IgG than IgM, which motivates for using IgG LFA readouts for serosurveys or home use.[33] Overall, FINDdx reports that most LFAs target the N antigen (see **Table 1**), making them more appropriate for testing breakthrough SARS-CoV-2 infections in individuals who received S-based vaccines.

Study Design to Evaluate Serologic Lateral Flow Assays

Decentralized administration of serologic tests raises important concerns about the accuracy of these platforms, subsequent interpretation of test results by both providers and end-users,[123] and their suitability for different implementation scenarios.[124] These considerations are summarized in **Table 2**.

STUDY POPULATION

It is important that cohorts used for LFA evaluations reflect the characteristics of the intended populations for implementation. For example, if the intended application is testing the longevity of vaccine-induced response, the study design should include control pre-vaccination samples, proximal post-vaccination samples to assess seroconversion (e.g., 1- and 2-week post-vaccination) and remote samples (e.g., 6 months or 1-year post-vaccination). In this situation, quantitative serologic assays such as ELISAs should be used as a reference to benchmark the LFA performance.[33] In contrast, if LFAs are intended to test the induction of antibodies in specific subgroups, such as HIV-positive or immunocompromised individuals,[125] the cohorts need to include individuals with these clinical characteristics and controls. In contrast, evaluation of LFA's analytical specificity against other related viruses will require inclusion of populations with a known history of exposure to other coronaviruses, such as historical samples from convalescent individuals from the first SARS-CoV epidemic in 2003,[126] as SARS-CoV and SARS-CoV-2 share 76.5% amino acid sequence similarity, and share tropism for the ACE2 receptors for entry into mammalian cells.[127]

Symptomatic SARS-CoV-2 infection increases the pretest probability that someone was exposed to SARS-CoV-2. However, as asymptomatic SARS-CoV-2 carriers are estimated to comprise at least 40% to 45% of all SARS-CoV-2 infected individuals,[128] evaluation studies should include both symptomatic, as well as asymptomatic individuals,[129] with a positive SARS-CoV-2 result on a highly sensitive and specific molecular test. These studies were difficult at the beginning of the pandemic as testing was generally restricted to hospitalized and severely ill patients with COVID-19. However, with expanded access to community testing using sensitive RT-qPCR tests, inclusion of SARS-CoV-2-positive individuals with mild or no symptoms for sampling to evaluate serologic LFAs is important. The cases should ideally span diverse demographics, clinical presentations (from asymptomatic, mildly, and severely symptomatic to those in intensive care), and comorbidities, which may compromise seroconversion following SARS-CoV-2 infection, especially that some of these populations may be at even higher risk of SARS-CoV-2 infection and COVID-19 disease.[130,131] The parallel uninfected controls should preferably be sampled from the same population as cases to reduce systematic biases in the evaluation.

The selection of SARS-CoV-2 unexposed controls is more difficult considering the wide-spread transmission of the virus and high seroprevalence globally.[2,5] The WHO only declared the pandemic a global emergency in March of 2020, whereas seroprevalence at these months indicated higher rates of infections that reflect earlier transmission.[132] Several communities outside of Wuhan already documented seropositive patients in January and February of 2020,[133] which may be due to cross-reactivity to other related coronaviruses, or real transmission of SARS-CoV-2 before molecular testing was widely implemented. Therefore, controls should be collected from earlier samples, even before October or November of 2019, to rule out unreported SARS-CoV-2 infection. One possible way to avoid including SARS-CoV-2 exposed individuals as negative controls is to use prepandemic bio-banked samples. Alternatively, individuals who are routinely tested for SARS-CoV-2, who have never had a positive test result would be the suitable "matched" uninfected group. This prospective evaluation of LFA effectiveness is especially critical as new variants circulate and may compromise the performance accuracy of the LFAs under evaluation.[134–136] However, in situations whereby controls are enrolled from the same SARS-CoV-2 exposed communities, repeat testing with highly sensitive molecular tests as well as complementary serologic tests that are more sensitive,[137] would be important to rule out prior exposure to the virus. This is particularly critical in prospective studies whereby LFAs are evaluated using freshly collected samples, such as whole blood from finger pricks or saliva.[104]

SAMPLING SCHEMES

In addition to the choice of the population of interest for LFA evaluation, the samples can either be collected cross-sectionally or longitudinally or using a hybrid of the 2 designs.[83,95] As above, the sampling scheme should address the intended use case. Evaluating LFAs to measure the durability of vaccine-induced antibodies will require longitudinal sampling,[138] whereas cross-sectional samples from confirmed SARS-CoV-2 exposed and unexposed individuals would suffice for the evaluation of LFAs for implementation in seroprevalence studies. For positive cases, samples should be collected at least 10 days[33] to 3 or more weeks[58] after symptom onset, for those with clear COVID-19 symptoms, to allow sufficient time for seroconversion.[74] Asymptomatic study participants should be diagnosed by positive RT-qPCR results using a sensitive molecular test. In general, very low sensitivity and higher variability in accuracy were reported for LFAs measuring IgM and IgG from samples collected within a week postsymptoms onset.[103] This is consistent with the often-delayed seroconversion in patients with COVID-19 which occurs around day 11 to 19 postsymptoms onset.[139] Consequently, additional effort is required to improve the sensitivity of these assays for early detection of antibodies following symptoms onset.

SAMPLE SIZE DETERMINATION

One of the biggest limitations with the initial FDA EUA process for the evaluation of COVID-19 diagnostics was the small number of clinical samples needed from confirmed SARS-CoV-2-infected individuals.[23] Initial evaluations included fewer than 100 SARS-CoV-2 positive cases, which would only detect extreme differences in the accuracy of diagnostic platforms.[23,32] This is particularly critical whereby the prevalence of SARS-CoV-2 infections in various communities is still relatively low, as lower prevalence reduces the positive predictive value (PPV) of these tests.[114] Sample sizes to ensure adequate power are inversely correlated with the effect size differences to be detected at a prespecified significance level.[140] Consequently, a larger sample size will be required to compare the performance of 2 LFAs with close sensitivity levels (ie, small effect size), than comparing 2 LFAs with poor and excellent sensitivities (ie, large effect size). Considering the initially limited sample sizes for LFA evaluations, it is critical to expand sample sizes to validate the performance of LFAs to increase the confidence of assay performance before rollout.

SAMPLE CHOICE

Unlike nasopharyngeal swab samples that are hard to collect and have variable quality,[141] serology assays rely on serum and/or plasma samples collected from whole blood that is drawn by widely standardized procedures. Therefore, it is conceivable that some samples tested by RT-qPCR turn negative or indeterminate because of the quality of the sample tested or RNA degradation, leading to false-negative classifications. Serology is less likely to be impacted by sample quality. Furthermore, saliva samples have been evaluated for serology, particularly for the induction of IgA responses, but they are not the norm for LFA evaluations.[141] As the success of a diagnostic test depends on the quality of the biological specimen tested, serologic assays are appealing alternative tests because of the reliability of samples needed.

PERFORMANCE CHARACTERISTICS

To evaluate the accuracy of LFAs, several performance metrics need to be assessed based on the intended use cases. These characteristics include sensitivity, specificity, PPV or precision, and negative predictive values (NPVs), inter and intra-operator reproducibility and finally, analytical sensitivity, also known as LoD.

Sensitivity refers to the proportion of positive cases, defined by a gold standard test like a SARS-CoV-2 RT-qPCR, that are detected accurately by the test. A highly sensitive test will detect most cases, usually at the expense of inaccurately over-diagnosing uninfected individuals as false positives, and hence can be used to rule out disease when negative. PCR tests generally fall in this category,[142] as they are prone to detect very low concentrations of residual SARS-CoV-2 RNA molecules weeks after infection. Highly sensitive PCR tests may also detect contaminating templates from the environment or in the test reagents, as reported for the Cepheid Xpert Xpress SARS-CoV-2 test.[143] In contrast, the sensitivity of serologic tests is confounded by other factors, including time since symptom onset, the immunocompetence of study participants, the reactivity of the antibodies from a given sample to the antigen, and the emerging variants of SARS-CoV-2. The sensitivity of some LFAs was evaluated in samples from hospitalized patients with COVID-19 in a case-control study design, which likely overestimated the sensitivity of these compared with the general population,[144] leading to spectrum bias, that is, reporting different accuracies in the evaluation cohort and target population.

Specificity is the proportion of SARS-CoV-2-negative samples, which are correctly detected as negative by the LFA. The specificity of LFAs is expected to be generally high and close to 100%.[33,58,83,103,105] False-positives results could be caused by SARS-CoV-2 LFA cross-reactivity of antibodies against other circulating coronaviruses,[92] or inaccurate definitions of SARS-CoV-2 negative samples with a false-negative RT-qPCR or rapid antigen test result.

PPV refers to the proportion of positive tests that are likely to correspond to a SARS-CoV-2-positive sample. Conversely, NPV is the proportion of negative tests that are likely to come from true SARS-CoV-2-negative samples. It is important to note that PPV and NPV are a function of both the accuracy of the test and the seroprevalence in each population. Low prevalence penalizes the PPV of diagnostic tests, whereby a positive result is more likely to be a false positive the lower the infection rates are in a given population.[114] Thus, test outcomes, especially in nonhealth care settings have to be interpreted with caution and with an understanding of the community transmission dynamics and test limitations.[123]

Analytical sensitivity or LoD refers to the minimum SARS-CoV-2-specific antibody titers that are detectable by the LFA. Quantitative platforms such as ELISAs can be used to establish the LoD for LFAs, by adding titrated amounts of serologic standards with known antibody titers, and running them concurrently on the ELISA, or other quantitative platforms, and the LFAs under evaluation. Since LFAs are intended to be qualitative, it is worth considering whether a positive band needs to be detected by the naked eye, or whether additional smartphone apps or instruments can detect faint bands that correspond to low antibody concentrations in the sample.[99] The LoD of LFAs is higher than known sensitive quantitative methods such as the ultrasensitive Single molecule array (SIMOA) platforms.[33,137,145] However, a high LoD reduces the chance of misusing LFAs to ascribe immunity passports to individuals with low antibody titers to conservatively prevent overestimation of seroprevalence, and herd immunity.[27,28] Finally, testing the reproducibility of test results run by the same operator multiple times (intraoperator reproducibility), or between different operators (interoperator reproducibility), as well as reproducibility across different reagent lots would instill confidence in the reliability of the manufacturing quality of the LFAs.

IMPACT OF EMERGING VARIANTS ON THE PERFORMANCE OF LATERAL FLOW ASSAYS

The emergence of SARS-CoV-2 variants is an important consideration in the evaluation of SARS-CoV-2 diagnostic tests, since SARS-CoV-2 antigenic drift may reduce the sensitivity of these tests.[146] So far, at least 3 known variants of SARS-CoV-2 have been described that are characterized by novel genetic mutations. These include B.1.1.7,[147] B.1.351,[148] and P.1 and P.2.[149] B.1.1.7 has 23 mutations located in the open reading frame (ORF)1ab, ORF8, and N regions. Out of the 23 mutations, 17 are of concern whereby 13 are nonsynonymous, resulting in amino acid substitutions, and 4 are deletions. B.1.351 has 21 mutations including 9 amino acid changes in the S gene. The other mutations are in ORF1ab, ORF3a, N, and E genes. The P.1 variant has 10 mutations in the S gene, with additional mutations in ORF1ab, ORF8, and N genes. These emerging SARS-CoV-2 variant strains have compromised the ability of naturally induced antibodies to neutralize SARS-CoV-2.[135] For example, a new SARS-CoV-2 variant, 501Y.V2, substantially or completely escapes from neutralizing antibodies in COVID-19 convalescent plasma.[150]

Variants of SARS-CoV-2 with the D614G mutation in the spike (S) protein that increases receptor-binding avidity have also been reported globally[151] (**Table 3**). The B.1.351 and B.1.1.28 (P.1) variants are known to affect the performance of real-time RT-qPCR tests.[151] Patients infected with the H69del/V70del SARS-CoV-2 variant have an increased Spike (S) protein gene amplification drop-out rate, which leads to RT-qPCR target failure.[152]

The mature SARS-CoV-2 Spike trimer is composed of the exterior S1 and transmembrane S2 subunits.[153] The S1 subunit uses the RBD to interact with the ACE2 receptor, whereas the S2 subunit governs the fusion between the viral and cellular membranes. Spike is considered the major target of the cellular and humoral responses against SARS-CoV-2 in natural infection.[84,96] Of all SARS-CoV-2 variants, the D614G mutant accounts for 75.7% of all circulating strains and is associated with severe clinical presentation.[153] SARS-CoV-2 Spike D614G had a more severe impact on antibody binding than the wild-type strain.[154] Studies using monoclonal antibodies (mAbs) have shown that V483A in the receptor-binding domain has a mutation frequency of more than 0.1%.[151] It showed decreased reactivity to the 2 mAbs (P2B-2F6 and X593) and the A475V is significantly resistant to several neutralizing antibodies.[151] Strains with combined D614G and I472V mutations have shown increased infectivity and more resistance to neutralizing antibodies.[151] Some variants, including

Table 3
Summary of emerging SARS-CoV-2 variants

	Variant Designation	Characteristic Mutations (Protein: Mutation) and Location
1	B.1.1.7 (20I/501Y.V1)	ORF1ab: T1001I, A1708D, I2230 T, del3675–3677 SGF S: del69–70 HV, del144Y, N501Y, A570D, D614G, P681H, T761I, S982A, D1118H ORF8: Q27stop, R52I, Y73C N: D3L, S235F
2	B.1.351 (20H/501Y.V2)	ORF1ab: K1655N E: P71L N: T205I S: K417N, E484K, N501Y, D614G, A701V
3	P.1 (20 J/501Y.V3)	ORF1ab: F681L, I760T, S1188L, K1795Q, del3675–3677 SGF, E5662D S: L18F, T20N, P26S, D138Y, R190S, K417T, E484K, N501Y, D614G, H655Y, T1027I ORF3a: C174G ORF8: E92K ORF9: Q77E ORF14: V49L N: P80R ORF1ab: F681L, I760T, S1188L, K1795Q, del3675–3677SGF, E5662D S: L18F, T20N, P26S, D138Y, R190S, K417T, E484K, N501Y, D614G, H655Y, T1027I ORF3a: C174G ORF8: E92K ORF9: Q77E ORF14: V49L N: P80R ORF1ab: F681L, I760T, S1188L, K1795Q, del3675–3677SGF, E5662D

N439K, L452R, A475V, V483A, F490L, and Y508H, do have decreased sensitivity to neutralizing mAbs.[151]

Most LFAs target the C-terminus of viral nucleocapsid (N) protein. B.1.1.7 mutations on the N gene are located at the N-terminus. Hence, this variant is unlikely to show an impact on LFA performance as the epitope for antibody recognition likely remained intact despite the mutation. Other LFAs target S protein coded by S gene, which recent data show has a majority of mutations, including spike mutation E484K that affect antibody response, and hence could affect the LFA performance. Collectively, whether these mutations reduce the sensitivity of LFAs needs to be systematically evaluated (**Table 4**).

Prospects for Next-Generation Lateral Flow Assays to Detect Severe Acute Respiratory Syndrome Coronavirus 2 Variants

To evaluate the detection of SARS-CoV-2 variant-specific antibodies, the mutated antigen from the variants should be included in the kit, especially when amino acid changes in the SARS-CoV-2 antigens are sufficient to alter antibody binding.[154] Hence, recombinant antigens reflecting the pseudotypes of the emerging variants should be incorporated in the next generations of LFAs. Subsequent evaluation efforts for LFAs should perhaps analyze both the conserved and mutated antigens to distinguish whether an infection has occurred and whether antibodies were generated in response to a mutant strain. It is important to note that the difference in antigenicity may be too subtle to influence the detection of antibody responses. However, as new SARS-CoV-2 variants are still emerging, it is imperative to iteratively develop and improve LFA assays to detect variant-specific serologic responses.

Table 4
The possible consequences of emerging SARS-CoV-2 mutations on LFA performance

Variant Designation	Impact on Performance of Rapid Lateral Flow Assays
B.1.1.7 (501Y.V1)	The N gene mutations in this variant are located at the N-terminal. An assessment by Public Health England found that five SARS-CoV-2 rapid antigen tests evaluated were all able to successfully detect the variant.[162] No evaluations were performed for serology LFAs.
B.1.351 (501Y.V2)	To date, no evaluation studies have been carried out to confirm that performance of serology LFAs is not affected, but no major performance deficits are anticipated.
P.1 (501Y.V3) and P.2	To date, no evaluation studies have been carried out to confirm that test performance is not affected, but no major performance deficits are anticipated.

Evaluation of Implementation Feasibility and Fitness for Use

Following the evaluation of the accuracy of LFAs, they need to be assessed for implementation effectiveness and fitness for use.[72,155] Effectiveness reflects whether the LFA is fit for implementation in the intended population and settings by evaluating relevant factors, including required storage conditions and affordability, particularly in resource-limited countries and communities.[4] For instance, if LFAs require refrigeration in hot regions with little access to stable electricity or testing in temperature-controlled settings as reported for rapid antigen LFAs,[156] they may not be fit for implementation in those contexts. It is also important to evaluate whether the kit manufacturers or governments have assumed the financial responsibility to ramp up the supply chain to avail the LFAs to communities. If communities assume the financial burden of evaluation and cost for large-scale implementation, it is unlikely that results would meaningfully improve the public health outcomes of these communities.

The WHO's standard for point-of-care tests, including LFAs, need to be ASSURED-"Affordable, Sensitive, Specific, User-friendly, Rapid and robust, Equipment-free and Deliverable to end-users".[157] Gaps in any of these criteria compromise the successful implementation of the evaluated LFAs, as previously reported for the diagnostics of sexually-transmitted infections.[158] Hence, if sustainable scale-up of LFAs is intended, then pilots for LFA design and implementation should consider "beginning with the end in mind" framework that enhances its potential for future large-scale impact.[159] For the successful programmatic implementation of LFAs in routine serosurveillance, the 13-step recommendation guide should be used:

1. Participatory stakeholder engagement to build ownership, generate political commitment, and create champions of LFAs.
2. Ensuring the product addresses relevant public health needs and that implementation is feasible.
3. Building stakeholder consensus on the contextual implication of scale-up.
4. Tailoring LFAs to diverse sociocultural and institutional settings to ensure early identification of both barriers and opportunities for scale-up.
5. Ensuring LFAs be as simple as possible for the ease of future scale-up in diverse populations.
6. The LFA should be tested in a variety of settings whereby scale-up is intended.
7. Testing of implementation appropriateness should include day-to-day situations, and resource-constrained health care settings.

8. The process of early implementation should be evaluated and documented using implementation research.
9. Advocacy for financial support from governments, donors, and funding agencies for scale-up and funding for transition from pilot to large-scale rollout.
10. Advocacy for review of policies, laws, and regulations to institutionalize LFAs at the national level and subsequent governance structures in countries.
11. Laying down structures that promote learning and dissemination of information.
12. Cautious, incremental, initial scale-up with appropriate documentation of the implementation pathway is crucial.
13. Compare the LFA to other published methods.

LFA evaluation studies should consider appropriate theoretic frameworks toward achieving adoption and sustainability. These should ideally guide evidence generation, contextualize implementation and facilitate iteration, adoption, and sustainability.

SUMMARY

In conclusion, serologic LFAs can be useful tools for estimating the true extent of SARS-CoV-2 globally, which is estimated considering inaccuracies in reporting, limited availability of molecular tests, and asymptomatic transmission. Due to their affordability and ease of implementation, LFAs can be crucial tools in determining appropriate public health mitigation responses against the COVID-19 pandemic. However, their deployment should be coupled by rigorous evaluation both for their accuracy and their fitness for implementation in a variety of health care and community settings and can guide critical decisions such as the opening of economies from the socially and economically disruptive nation-wide lockdown measures. LFAs should also be evaluated in the context of vaccine rollouts and emerging variants.

CLINICS CARE POINTS

- Serological tests to monitor anti-SARS-CoV-2 antibodies, including LFAs, are better suited for population surveillance and research studies to monitor the longevity of infection- or vaccine-induced antibody responses. However, they are not well-suited to inform clincial decisions at the individual level, since their performance relies on several characteristics, which impact their positive and negative predictive values.

ACKNOWLEDGMENTS

S. Suliman is funded by a grant from Massachusetts Life Sciences Center (Accelerating Coronavirus Testing Solutions). J. Gitaka is funded by the African Academy of Sciences (Grants numbers GCA/MNCH/Round8/207/008 and SARSCov2-4-20-010) and the Royal Society, UK, Grant number FLR\R1\201314. L. Ochola is funded by the African Research Network for Neglected Tropical Diseases (ARNTD) small grants program Reference SGPIII/0210/351.

REFERENCES:

1. Chauhan V, Galwankar SC, Yellapu V, et al. State of the globe: the trials and tribulations of the COVID-19 pandemic: Separated but together, telemedicine revolution, frontline Struggle against "Silent Hypoxia," the relentless Search for

    novel therapeutics and vaccines, and the daunting prospect of "COVIFLU". J Glob Infect Dis 2020;12(2):39–43.

2. Dong E, Du H, Gardner L. An interactive web-based dashboard to track COVID-19 in real time. Lancet Infect Dis 2020;20(5):533–4.

3. Kumar R, Nagpal S, Kaushik S, et al. COVID-19 diagnostic approaches: different roads to the same destination. Virusdisease 2020;31(2):97–105.

4. Peeling RW, Wedderburn CJ, Garcia PJ, et al. Serology testing in the COVID-19 pandemic response. Lancet Infect Dis 2020;20(9):e245–9.

5. Arora RK, Joseph A, Van Wyk J, et al. SeroTracker: a global SARS-CoV-2 sero-prevalence dashboard. Lancet Infect Dis 2021;21(4):e75–6.

6. Aschwanden C. Five reasons why COVID herd immunity is probably impossible. Nature 2021;591(7851):520–2.

7. Kissler SM, Tedijanto C, Goldstein E, et al. Projecting the transmission dynamics of SARS-CoV-2 through the postpandemic period. Science 2020;368(6493):860–8.

8. Saffary T, Adegboye OA, Gayawan E, et al. Analysis of COVID-19 cases' Spatial dependence in US counties reveals health inequalities. Front Public Health 2020;8:579190.

9. Tan TQ, Kullar R, Swartz TH, et al. Location matters: geographic disparities and impact of coronavirus disease 2019. J Infect Dis 2020;222(12):1951–4.

10. Yamey G, Schaferhoff M, Hatchett R, et al. Ensuring global access to COVID-19 vaccines. Lancet 2020;395(10234):1405–6.

11. Shaw JA, Meiring M, Cummins T, et al. Higher SARS-CoV-2 seroprevalence in workers with lower socioeconomic status in Cape Town, South Africa. PLoS One 2021;16(2):e0247852.

12. Batchi-Bouyou AL, Lobaloba L, Ndounga M, et al. High SARS-COV2 IgG/IGM seroprevalence in asymptomatic Congolese in Brazzaville, the republic of Congo. Int J Infect Dis 2020;106:3–7.

13. George CE, Inbaraj LR, Chandrasingh S, et al. High seroprevalence of COVID-19 infection in a large slum in South India; what does it tell us about managing a pandemic and beyond? Epidemiol Infect 2021;149:e39.

14. Arevalo-Rodriguez I, Seron P, Buitrago-Garcia D, et al. Recommendations for SARS-CoV-2/COVID-19 testing: a scoping review of current guidance. BMJ Open 2021;11(1):e043004.

15. Tahmasebi S, Khosh E, Esmaeilzadeh A. The outlook for diagnostic purposes of the 2019-novel coronavirus disease. J Cell Physiol 2020;235(12):9211–29.

16. Long QX, Liu BZ, Deng HJ, et al. Antibody responses to SARS-CoV-2 in patients with COVID-19. Nat Med 2020;26(6):845–8.

17. Theel ES, Slev P, Wheeler S, et al. The role of antibody testing for SARS-CoV-2: is there one? J Clin Microbiol 2020;58(8). e00797-20.

18. Hellou MM, Gorska A, Mazzaferri F, et al. Nucleic-acid-amplification tests from respiratory samples for the diagnosis of coronavirus infections: systematic review and meta-analysis. Clin Microbiol Infect 2021;27(3):341–51.

19. Toptan T, Eckermann L, Pfeiffer AE, et al. Evaluation of a SARS-CoV-2 rapid antigen test: potential to help reduce community spread? J Clin Virol 2021;135:104713.

20. Pilarowski G, Lebel P, Sunshine S, et al. Performance characteristics of a rapid SARS-CoV-2 antigen detection assay at a public plaza testing site in San Francisco. J Infect Dis 2021. https://doi.org/10.1101/2020.11.02.20223891.

21. Pollock NR, Jacobs JR, Tran K, et al. Performance and implementation evaluation of the Abbott BinaxNOW rapid antigen test in a high-throughput drive-

through community testing site in Massachusetts. J Clin Microbiol 2021;59(5). e00083-21.

22. Deeks JJ, Dinnes J, Takwoingi Y, et al. Antibody tests for identification of current and past infection with SARS-CoV-2. Cochrane Database Syst Rev 2020;6: CD013652.

23. FDA. EUA authorized serology test performance. United States Food and Drug administration. 2020. Available at: https://www.fda.gov/medical-devices/coronavirus-disease-2019-covid-19-emergency-use-authorizations-medical-devices/eua-authorized-serology-test-performance. Accessed December 25, 2020.

24. Badnjevic A, Pokvic LG, Dzemic Z, et al. Risks of emergency use authorizations for medical products during outbreak situations: a COVID-19 case study. Biomed Eng Online 2020;19(1):75.

25. Lisboa Bastos M, Tavaziva G, Abidi SK, et al. Diagnostic accuracy of serological tests for covid-19: systematic review and meta-analysis. BMJ 2020;370:m2516.

26. Page M, Almond N, Rose NJ, et al. Diagnostics and the coronavirus: don't let the standards slip. Nat Biotechnol 2020;38(6):673-4.

27. Brown RCH, Kelly D, Wilkinson D, et al. The scientific and ethical feasibility of immunity passports. Lancet Infect Dis 2020;21(3):e58-63.

28. Waller J, Rubin GJ, Potts HWW, et al. Immunity Passports' for SARS-CoV-2: an online experimental study of the impact of antibody test terminology on perceived risk and behaviour. BMJ Open 2020;10(8):e040448.

29. WHO. "Immunity passports" in the context of COVID-19. World Health Organization commentaries. 2020. Available at: https://www.who.int/news-room/commentaries/detail/immunity-passports-in-the-context-of-covid-19. Accessed December 25, 2020.

30. WHO. Population-based age-stratified seroepidemiological investigation protocol for COVID-19 virus infection. Available at: https://appswhoint/iris/handle/10665/331656 2020. Accessed May 18, 2020.

31. World Health Organization. (↱2020)↱. Diagnostic testing for SARS-CoV-2: interim guidance, 11 September 2020. World Health Organization. Available at: https://apps.who.int/iris/handle/10665/334254. License: CC BY-NC-SA 3.0 IGO.

32. FIND. FIND (foundation for innovative new diagnostics) evaluation update: SARS-CoV-2 immunoassays. Access to COVID-19 tools (ACT) Accelerator. 2020. Available at: https://www.finddx.org/sarscov2-eval-antibody/. Accessed March 28, 2021.

33. Bianca A, Trombetta SEK, Kitchen RR, et al. Evaluation of serological lateral flow assays for severe acute respiratory syndrome coronavirus-2. BMC Infect Dis 2021;21(1):580. https://doi.org/10.1186/s12879-021-06257-7.

34. Ling R, Yu Y, He J, et al. Seroprevalence and epidemiological characteristics of immunoglobulin M and G antibodies against SARS-CoV-2 in asymptomatic people in Wuhan, China: a cross-sectional study. BioRxiv 2020. https://doi.org/10.1101/2020.06.16.20132423. Available at: https://www.medrxiv.org/content/10.1101/2020.06.16.20132423v3.article-info.

35. Xu X, Sun J, Nie S, et al. Seroprevalence of immunoglobulin M and G antibodies against SARS-CoV-2 in China. Nat Med 2020;26(8):1193-5.

36. Rogawski McQuade ET, Guertin KA, Becker L, et al. Assessment of seroprevalence of SARS-CoV-2 and risk factors associated with COVID-19 infection among outpatients in Virginia. JAMA Netw Open 2021;4(2):e2035234.

37. Bajema KL, Wiegand RE, Cuffe K, et al. Estimated SARS-CoV-2 seroprevalence in the US as of September 2020. JAMA Intern Med 2020;181(4):450–60.

38. Mahase E. Covid-19: antibody prevalence in England fell from 6.0% to 4.4% over three months, study finds. BMJ 2020;371:m4163.

39. Galan MI, Velasco M, Casas ML, et al. Hospital-Wide SARS-CoV-2 seropreva-lence in health care workers in a Spanish teaching hospital. Enferm Infecc Mi-crobiol Clin 2020. https://doi.org/10.1016/j.eimc.2020.11.015.

40. Nisar MI, Ansari N, Khalid F, et al. Serial population-based sero-surveys for COVID-19 in two neighborhoods of Karachi, Pakistan. Int J Infect Dis 2021; 106:176–82.

41. Verani A, Clodfelter C, Menon AN, et al. Social distancing policies in 22 African countries during the COVID-19 pandemic: a desk review. Pan Afr Med J 2020; 37(Suppl 1):46.

42. Lalaoui R, Bakour S, Raoult D, et al. What could explain the late emergence of COVID-19 in Africa? New Microbes New Infect 2020;38:100760.

43. Rice BL, Annapragada A, Baker RE, et al. Variation in SARS-CoV-2 outbreaks across sub-Saharan Africa. Nat Med 2021;27(3):447–53.

44. Post LA, Argaw ST, Jones C, et al. A SARS-CoV-2 surveillance System in sub-Saharan Africa: modeling study for persistence and transmission to inform pol-icy. J Med Internet Res 2020;22(11):e24248.

45. Diop BZ, Ngom M, Pougue Biyong C, et al. The relatively young and rural pop-ulation may limit the spread and severity of COVID-19 in Africa: a modelling study. BMJ Glob Health 2020;5(5):e002699.

46. Uyoga S, Adetifa IMO, Karanja HK, et al. Seroprevalence of anti-SARS-CoV-2 IgG antibodies in Kenyan blood donors. Science 2021;371(6524):79–82.

47. Lucinde R, Mugo D, Bottomley C, et al. Sero-surveillance for IgG to SARS-CoV-2 at antenatal care clinics in two Kenyan referral hospitals. MedRxiv 2021. https://doi.org/10.1101/2021.02.05.21250735. Available at: https://www.medrxiv.org/content/10.1101/2021.02.05.21250735v1.

48. Chibwana MG, Jere KC, Kamng'ona R, et al. High SARS-CoV-2 seroprevalence in Health Care Workers but relatively low numbers of deaths in urban Malawi. Wellcome Open Research 2021. https://doi.org/10.12688/wellcomeopenres.16188.1.

49. Kempen JH, Abashawl A, Suga HK, et al. SARS-CoV-2 serosurvey in Addis Ababa, Ethiopia. Am J Trop Med Hyg 2020;103(5):2022–3.

50. Olayanju O, Bamidele O, Edem F, et al. SARS-CoV-2 Seropositivity in asymp-tomatic frontline health workers in ibadan, Nigeria. Am J Trop Med Hyg 2021; 104(1):91–4.

51. Benn CS, Salinha A, Mendes S, et al. SARS-CoV2 sero-survey among adults involved in health care and health research in Guinea-Bissau, West Africa. MedRxiv 2021. https://doi.org/10.1101/2021.03.06.21253046. Available at: https://www.medrxiv.org/content/10.1101/2021.03.06.21253046v1.

52. Wiens KE, Mawien PN, Rumunu J, et al. Seroprevalence of anti-SARS-CoV-2 IgG antibodies in Juba, South Sudan: a population-based study. Emerg Infect Dis 2021;27(6):1598–606. https://doi.org/10.3201/eid2706.210568.

53. Bobrovitz N, Arora RK, Yan T, et al. Lessons from a rapid systematic review of early SARS-CoV-2 serosurveys. MedRxiv 2020. https://doi.org/10.1101/2020.05.10.20097451. Available at: https://www.medrxiv.org/content/10.1101/2020.05.10.20097451v1.

54. McCreesh N, Dlamini V, Edwards A, et al. Impact of social distancing regula-tions and epidemic risk perception on social contact and SARS-CoV-2

transmission potential in rural South Africa: analysis of repeated cross-sectional surveys. BMC Infect Dis 2021;21(1):928. https://doi.org/10.1186/s12879-021-06604-8.

55. LeBlanc EV, Colpitts CC. A dual antibody test for accurate surveillance of SARS-CoV-2 exposure rates. Cell Rep Med 2021;2(3):100223.

56. D'Cruz RJ, Currier AW, Sampson VB. Laboratory testing methods for novel severe acute respiratory syndrome-coronavirus-2 (SARS-CoV-2). Front Cell Dev Biol 2020;8:468.

57. Pickering S, Betancor G, Galao RP, et al. Comparative assessment of multiple COVID-19 serological technologies supports continued evaluation of point-of-care lateral flow assays in hospital and community healthcare settings. Plos Pathog 2020;16(9):e1008817.

58. Whitman JD, Hiatt J, Mowery CT, et al. Evaluation of SARS-CoV-2 serology assays reveals a range of test performance. Nat Biotechnol 2020;38(10):1174–83.

59. Miller TE, Garcia Beltran WF, Bard AZ, et al. Clinical sensitivity and interpretation of PCR and serological COVID-19 diagnostics for patients presenting to the hospital. FASEB J 2020;34(10):13877–84.

60. Roy V, Fischinger S, Atyeo C, et al. SARS-CoV-2-specific ELISA development. J Immunol Methods 2020;484-485:112832.

61. Zhong L, Chuan J, Gong B, et al. Detection of serum IgM and IgG for COVID-19 diagnosis. Sci China Life Sci 2020;63(5):777–80.

62. Van Elslande J, Houben E, Depypere M, et al. Diagnostic performance of seven rapid IgG/IgM antibody tests and the Euroimmun IgA/IgG ELISA in COVID-19 patients. Clin Microbiol Infect 2020;26(8):1082–7.

63. Okba NMA, Muller MA, Li W, et al. Severe acute respiratory syndrome coronavirus 2-specific antibody responses in coronavirus disease patients. Emerg Infect Dis 2020;26(7):1478–88.

64. Beavis KG, Matushek SM, Abeleda APF, et al. Evaluation of the EUROIMMUN anti-SARS-CoV-2 ELISA assay for detection of IgA and IgG antibodies. J Clin Virol 2020;129:104468.

65. Tre-Hardy M, Wilmet A, Beukinga I, et al. Analytical and clinical validation of an ELISA for specific SARS-CoV-2 IgG, IgA, and IgM antibodies. J Med Virol 2021;93(2):803–11.

66. Sapkal G, Shete-Aich A, Jain R, et al. Development of indigenous IgG ELISA for the detection of anti-SARS-CoV-2 IgG. Indian J Med Res 2020;151(5):444–9.

67. Alandijany TA, El-Kafrawy SA, Tolah AM, et al. Development and Optimization of in-house ELISA for detection of human IgG antibody to SARS-CoV-2 full Length spike protein. Pathogens 2020;9(10):803.

68. Brochot E, Demey B, Touze A, et al. Anti-spike, anti-nucleocapsid and neutralizing antibodies in SARS-CoV-2 inpatients and asymptomatic individuals. Front Microbiol 2020;11:584251.

69. Weber MC, Risch M, Thiel SL, et al. Characteristics of three different chemiluminescence assays for testing for SARS-CoV-2 antibodies. Dis Markers 2021;2021:8810196.

70. Pecora ND, Zand MS. Measuring the serologic response to severe acute respiratory syndrome coronavirus 2: methods and meaning. Clin Lab Med 2020;40(4):603–14.

71. Ragnesola B, Jin D, Lamb CC, et al. COVID19 antibody detection using lateral flow assay tests in a cohort of convalescent plasma donors. BMC Res Notes 2020;13(1):372.

72. Humble RM, Merrill AE, Ford BA, et al. Practical considerations for implementation of SARS-CoV-2 serological testing in the clinical laboratory: Experience at an Academic medical center. Acad Pathol 2021;8. 23742895211002802.

73. Lou B, Li TD, Zheng SF, et al. Serology characteristics of SARS-CoV-2 infection after exposure and post-symptom onset. Eur Respir J 2020;56(2):2000763.

74. Zhao J, Yuan Q, Wang H, et al. Antibody responses to SARS-CoV-2 in patients with novel coronavirus disease 2019. Clin Infect Dis 2020;71(16):2027–34.

75. Sette A, Crotty S. Adaptive immunity to SARS-CoV-2 and COVID-19. Cell 2021; 184(4):861–80.

76. Jarjour NN, Masopust D, Jameson SC. T cell memory: understanding COVID-19. Immunity 2021;54(1):14–8.

77. Ni L, Ye F, Cheng ML, et al. Detection of SARS-CoV-2-specific humoral and cellular immunity in COVID-19 convalescent individuals. Immunity 2020;52(6): 971–7.e3.

78. Yu KK, Fischinger S, Smith MT, et al. Comorbid illnesses are associated with altered adaptive immune responses to SARS-CoV-2. JCI Insight 2021;6(6): e146242.

79. Yu KKQ, Fischinger S, Smith MT, et al. Comorbid illnesses are associated with altered adaptive immune responses to SARS-CoV-2. JCI Insight 2021;6(6): e146242. https://doi.org/10.1172/jci.insight.146242.

80. Ali MG, Zhang Z, Gao Q, et al. Recent advances in therapeutic applications of neutralizing antibodies for virus infections: an overview. Immunol Res 2020; 68(6):325–39.

81. Tian X, Li C, Huang A, et al. Potent binding of 2019 novel coronavirus spike protein by a SARS coronavirus-specific human monoclonal antibody. Emerg Microbes Infect 2020;9(1):382–5.

82. Krishnamurthy HK, Jayaraman V, Krishna K, et al. Antibody profiling and prevalence in US patients during the SARS-CoV2 pandemic. PLoS One 2020; 15(11):e0242655.

83. Post N, Eddy D, Huntley C, et al. Antibody response to SARS-CoV-2 infection in humans: a systematic review. PLoS One 2020;15(12):e0244126.

84. Premkumar L, Segovia-Chumbez B, Jadi R, et al. The receptor binding domain of the viral spike protein is an immunodominant and highly specific target of antibodies in SARS-CoV-2 patients. Sci Immunol 2020;5(48):eabc8413.

85. Hoffmann M, Kleine-Weber H, Schroeder S, et al. SARS-CoV-2 cell entry depends on ACE2 and TMPRSS2 and is blocked by a clinically proven protease inhibitor. Cell 2020;181(2):271–80.e8.

86. Bourgonje AR, Abdulle AE, Timens W, et al. Angiotensin-converting enzyme 2 (ACE2), SARS-CoV-2 and the pathophysiology of coronavirus disease 2019 (COVID-19). J Pathol 2020;251(3):228–48.

87. Dejnirattisai W, Zhou D, Ginn HM, et al. The antigenic anatomy of SARS-CoV-2 receptor binding domain. Cell 2021;184(8):2183–200.e22.

88. Amanat F, Stadlbauer D, Strohmeier S, et al. A serological assay to detect SARS-CoV-2 seroconversion in humans. Nat Med 2020;26(7):1033–6.

89. Corbett KS, Edwards DK, Leist SR, et al. SARS-CoV-2 mRNA vaccine design enabled by prototype pathogen preparedness. Nature 2020;586(7830):567–71.

90. Sethuraman N, Jeremiah SS, Ryo A. Interpreting diagnostic tests for SARS-CoV-2. JAMA 2020;323(22):2249–51.

91. Bryan A, Pepper G, Wener MH, et al. Performance characteristics of the Abbott Architect SARS-CoV-2 IgG assay and seroprevalence in Boise, Idaho. J Clin Microbiol 2020;58(8). e00941-20.

92. Anderson EM, Goodwin EC, Verma A, et al. Seasonal human coronavirus antibodies are boosted upon SARS-CoV-2 infection but not associated with protection. Cell 2021;184(7):1858–64.e10.

93. Krammer F, Simon V. Serology assays to manage COVID-19. Science 2020; 368(6495):1060–1.

94. Michel M, Bouam A, Edouard S, et al. Evaluating ELISA, immunofluorescence, and lateral flow assay for SARS-CoV-2 serologic assays. Front Microbiol 2020; 11:597529.

95. He Z, Ren L, Yang J, et al. Seroprevalence and humoral immune durability of anti-SARS-CoV-2 antibodies in Wuhan, China: a longitudinal, population-level, cross-sectional study. Lancet 2021;397(10279):1075–84.

96. Iyer AS, Jones FK, Nodoushani A, et al. Persistence and decay of human antibody responses to the receptor binding domain of SARS-CoV-2 spike protein in COVID-19 patients. Sci Immunol 2020;5(52):eabe0367.

97. Ernst E, Wolfe P, Stahura C, et al. Technical considerations to development of serological tests for SARS-CoV-2. Talanta 2021;224:121883.

98. Cavalera S, Colitti B, Rosati S, et al. A multi-target lateral flow immunoassay enabling the specific and sensitive detection of total antibodies to SARS COV-2. Talanta 2021;223(Pt 1):121737.

99. Roda A, Cavalera S, Di Nardo F, et al. Dual lateral flow optical/chemiluminescence immunosensors for the rapid detection of salivary and serum IgA in patients with COVID-19 disease. Biosens Bioelectron 2021;172:112765.

100. Li Z, Yi Y, Luo X, et al. Development and clinical application of a rapid IgM-IgG combined antibody test for SARS-CoV-2 infection diagnosis. J Med Virol 2020; 92(9):1518–24.

101. Calabria D, Caliceti C, Zangheri M, et al. Smartphone-based enzymatic biosensor for oral fluid L-lactate detection in one minute using confined multilayer paper reflectometry. Biosens Bioelectron 2017;94:124–30.

102. Neagu M. The bumpy road to achieve herd immunity in COVID-19. J Immunoassay Immunochem 2020;1–18.

103. Hashem AM, Alhabbab RY, Algaissi A, et al. Performance of commercially available rapid serological assays for the detection of SARS-CoV-2 antibodies. Pathogens 2020;9(12):1067.

104. Singh NK, Ray P, Carlin AF, et al. Hitting the diagnostic sweet spot: point-of-care SARS-CoV-2 salivary antigen testing with an off-the-shelf glucometer. Biosens Bioelectron 2021;180:113111.

105. Lee W, Straube S, Sincic R, et al. Clinical evaluation of a COVID-19 antibody lateral flow assay using point of care samples. medRxiv 2020. https://doi.org/10.1101/2020.12.02.20242750.

106. Nilsson AC, Holm DK, Justesen US, et al. Comparison of six commercially available SARS-CoV-2 antibody assays-Choice of assay depends on intended use. Int J Infect Dis 2021;103:381–8.

107. Ibarrondo FJ, Fulcher JA, Goodman-Meza D, et al. Rapid decay of anti-SARS-CoV-2 antibodies in persons with mild covid-19. N Engl J Med 2020;383(11): 1085–7.

108. Iwasaki A, Yang Y. The potential danger of suboptimal antibody responses in COVID-19. Nat Rev Immunol 2020;20(6):339–41.

109. Niu Y, Xu F. Deciphering the power of isolation in controlling COVID-19 outbreaks. Lancet Glob Health 2020;8(4):e452–3.

110. Jorfi M, Luo NM, Hazra A, et al. Diagnostic technology for COVID-19: comparative evaluation of antigen and serology-based SARS-CoV-2 immunoassays,

and contact tracing solutions for potential use as at-home products. MedRxiv 2020. https://doi.org/10.1101/2020.06.25.20140236.

111. Ravi N, Cortade DL, Ng E, et al. Diagnostics for SARS-CoV-2 detection: a comprehensive review of the FDA-EUA COVID-19 testing landscape. Biosens Bioelectron 2020;165:112454.

112. IndustryPlaybook. Gauss and Cellex partner for first at-home SARS-CoV-2 antigen test. Clinical laboratory news. 2020. Available at: https://www.aacc.org/cln/articles/2020/november/gauss-and-cellex-partner-for-first-at-home-sars-cov-2-antigen-test. Accessed April 12, 2020.

113. Choudhary MC, Crain CR, Qiu X, et al. SARS-CoV-2 sequence characteristics of COVID-19 persistence and reinfection. Clin Infect Dis 2021. https://doi.org/10.1093/cid/ciab380.

114. Tenny S, Hoffman MR. Prevalence. In: . Treasure Island (FL): StatPearls; 2020.

115. Garritsen A, Scholzen A, van den Nieuwenhof DWA, et al. Two-tiered SARS-CoV-2 seroconversion screening in The Netherlands and stability of nucleocapsid, spike protein domain 1 and neutralizing antibodies. Infect Dis (Lond) 2021; 53(7):498–512.

116. Lan J, Ge J, Yu J, et al. Structure of the SARS-CoV-2 spike receptor-binding domain bound to the ACE2 receptor. Nature 2020;581(7807):215–20.

117. Jackson LA, Anderson EJ, Rouphael NG, et al. An mRNA vaccine against SARS-CoV-2 - preliminary report. N Engl J Med 2020;383(20):1920–31.

118. Voysey M, Clemens SAC, Madhi SA, et al. Safety and efficacy of the ChAdOx1 nCoV-19 vaccine (AZD1222) against SARS-CoV-2: an interim analysis of four randomised controlled trials in Brazil, South Africa, and the UK. Lancet 2021; 397(10269):99–111.

119. Mercado NB, Zahn R, Wegmann F, et al. Single-shot Ad26 vaccine protects against SARS-CoV-2 in rhesus macaques. Nature 2020;586(7830):583–8.

120. Polack FP, Thomas SJ, Kitchin N, et al. Safety and efficacy of the BNT162b2 mRNA covid-19 vaccine. N Engl J Med 2020;383(27):2603–15.

121. Thiagarajan K. What do we know about India's Covaxin vaccine? BMJ 2021;373: n997.

122. Suhandynata RT, Bevins NJ, Tran JT, et al. SARS-CoV-2 serology status detected by commercialized platforms distinguishes previous infection and vaccination adaptive immune responses. J Appl Lab Med 2021;6(5):1109–22. https://doi.org/10.1093/jalm/jfab080.

123. Syal K. Guidelines on newly identified limitations of diagnostic tools for COVID-19 and consequences. J Med Virol 2021;93(4):1837–42.

124. Kirk MA, Kelley C, Yankey N, et al. A systematic review of the use of the consolidated framework for implementation research. Implement Sci 2016;11:72.

125. Choi B, Choudhary MC, Regan J, et al. Persistence and evolution of SARS-CoV-2 in an immunocompromised host. N Engl J Med 2020;383(23):2291–3.

126. Zhu Y, Yu D, Han Y, et al. Cross-reactive neutralization of SARS-CoV-2 by serum antibodies from recovered SARS patients and immunized animals. Sci Adv 2020;6(45):eabc9999.

127. Wang H, Li X, Li T, et al. The genetic sequence, origin, and diagnosis of SARS-CoV-2. Eur J Clin Microbiol Infect Dis 2020;39(9):1629–35.

128. Oran DP, Topol EJ. Prevalence of asymptomatic SARS-CoV-2 infection : a Narrative review. Ann Intern Med 2020;173(5):362–7.

129. Milani GP, Dioni L, Favero C, et al. Serological follow-up of SARS-CoV-2 asymptomatic subjects. Sci Rep 2020;10(1):20048.

130. Kullar R, Marcelin JR, Swartz TH, et al. Racial disparity of coronavirus disease 2019 in African American communities. J Infect Dis 2020;222(6):890–3.
131.. Menezes NP, Malone J, Lyons C, et al. Racial and Ethnic disparities in viral acute respiratory infections in the United States: protocol of a systematic review. Syst Rev 2021;10(1):196. https://doi.org/10.1186/s13643-021-01749-8.
132. To KK, Cheng VC, Cai JP, et al. Seroprevalence of SARS-CoV-2 in Hong Kong and in residents evacuated from Hubei province, China: a multicohort study. Lancet Microbe 2020;1(3):e111–8.
133. Haveri A, Smura T, Kuivanen S, et al. Serological and molecular findings during SARS-CoV-2 infection: the first case study in Finland, January to February 2020. Euro Surveill 2020;25(11):2000266. https://doi.org/10.2807/1560-7917.ES.2020.25.11.2000266.
134. Poterico JA, Mestanza O. Genetic variants and source of introduction of SARS-CoV-2 in South America. J Med Virol 2020;92(10):2139–45.
135. Chen R, Xie X, Case J, et al. SARS-CoV-2 variants show resistance to neutralization by many monoclonal and serum-derived polyclonal antibodies. Nat Med 2021;27(4):717–26. https://doi.org/10.1038/s41591-021-01294-w.
136. Wibmer CK, Ayres F, Hermanus T, et al. SARS-CoV-2 501Y.V2 escapes neutralization by South African COVID-19 donor plasma. Nat Med 2021;27(4):622–5.
137. Norman M, Gilboa T, Ogata AF, et al. Ultrasensitive high-resolution profiling of early seroconversion in patients with COVID-19. Nat Biomed Eng 2020;4(12):1180–7.
138. Widge AT, Rouphael NG, Jackson LA, et al. Durability of responses after SARS-CoV-2 mRNA-1273 vaccination. N Engl J Med 2021;384(1):80–2.
139. Hoffman T, Nissen K, Krambrich J, et al. Evaluation of a COVID-19 IgM and IgG rapid test; an efficient tool for assessment of past exposure to SARS-CoV-2. Infect Ecol Epidemiol 2020;10(1):1754538.
140. Krzywinski M, Altman N. Power and sample size. Nat Methods 2013;10(12):2.
141. Griesemer SB, Van Slyke G, Ehrbar D, et al. Evaluation of specimen types and saliva stabilization solutions for SARS-CoV-2 testing. J Clin Microbiol 2021;59(5). e01418-20.
142. Lorentzen HF, Schmidt SA, Sandholdt H, et al. Estimation of the diagnostic accuracy of real-time reverse transcription quantitative polymerase chain reaction for SARS-CoV-2 using re-analysis of published data. Dan Med J 2020;67(9). A04200237.
143. Falasca F, Sciandra I, Di Carlo D, et al. Detection of SARS-COV N2 Gene: very low amounts of viral RNA or false positive? J Clin Virol 2020;133:104660.
144. Takahashi S, Greenhouse B, Rodriguez-Barraquer I. Are seroprevalence estimates for severe acute respiratory syndrome coronavirus 2 biased? J Infect Dis 2020;222(11):1772–5.
145. Nilles EJ, Karlson EW, Norman M, et al. Evaluation of two commercial and two non-commercial immunoassays for the detection of prior infection to SARS-CoV-2. J Appl Lab Med 2021;6(6):1561–70. https://doi.org/10.1093/jalm/jfab072.
146. Yuan M, Huang D, Lee CD, et al. Structural and functional ramifications of antigenic drift in recent SARS-CoV-2 variants. Science 2021;373(6556):818–23. https://doi.org/10.1126/science.abh1139.
147. Leung K, Shum MH, Leung GM, et al. Early transmissibility assessment of the N501Y mutant strains of SARS-CoV-2 in the United Kingdom, October to November 2020. Euro Surveill 2021;26(1):2002106.

148. Novazzi F, Genoni A, Spezia PG, et al. Introduction of SARS-CoV-2 variant of concern 20h/501Y.V2 (B.1.351) from Malawi to Italy. Emerg Microbes Infect 2021;10(1):710–2.
149. Maggi F, Novazzi F, Genoni A, et al. Imported SARS-CoV-2 variant P.1 in traveler returning from Brazil to Italy. Emerg Infect Dis 2021;27(4):1249–51.
150. Wibmer CK, Ayres F, Hermanus T, et al. SARS-CoV-2 501Y.V2 escapes neutralization by South African COVID-19 donor plasma. Nat Med 2021;27(4):622–5. https://doi.org/10.1038/s41591-021-01285-x.
151. Galloway SE, Paul P, MacCannell DR, et al. Emergence of SARS-CoV-2 B.1.1.7 Lineage - United States, december 29, 2020-January 12, 2021. MMWR Morb Mortal Wkly Rep 2021;70(3):95–9.
152. Washington NL, White S, Barrett KMS, et al. S gene dropout patterns in SARS-CoV-2 tests suggest spread of the H69del/V70del mutation in the US. MedRxiv 2020. https://doi.org/10.1101/2020.12.24.20248814. Available at: https://www.medrxiv.org/content/10.1101/2020.12.24.20248814v1.
153. Li Q, Wu J, Nie J, et al. The impact of mutations in SARS-CoV-2 spike on viral infectivity and antigenicity. Cell 2020;182(5):1284–94.e9.
154. Martin S, Heslan C, Jégou G, et al. SARS-CoV2 envelop proteins reshape the serological responses of COVID-19 patients. iScience 2021;24(10):103185. https://doi.org/10.1016/j.isci.2021.103185.
155. Huggett JF, Moran-Gilad J, Lee JE. COVID-19 new diagnostics development: novel detection methods for SARS-CoV-2 infection and considerations for their translation to routine use. Curr Opin Pulm Med 2021;27(3):155–62.
156. Haage V, Ferreira de Oliveira-Filho E, Moreira-Soto A, et al. Impaired performance of SARS-CoV-2 antigen-detecting rapid diagnostic tests at elevated and low temperatures. J Clin Virol 2021;138:104796.
157. Kosack CS, Page A, Klatser PR. A guide to aid the selection of diagnostic tests. Bull World Health Organ 2017;95(Policy and Practice):7.
158. WHO. Mapping the landscape of diagnostics for sexually transmitted infections: key findings and recommendations. World Health Organization; 2004. UNICEF/UNDP/World Bank/WHO Special Programme for Training in Tropical Diseases (TDR). Available at: https://www.who.int/tdr/publications/documents/mapping-landscape-sti.pdf.
159. World Health Organization. Beginning with the end in mind: planning pilot projects and other programmatic research for successful scaling up, 2011. World Health Organization. Available at: http://apps.who.int/iris/bitstream/handle/10665/44708/9789241502320_eng.pdf;jsessionid=20930C5E4214A2F58 3E331724B127B14?sequence=1.
160. Proctor E, Silmere H, Raghavan R, et al. Outcomes for implementation research: conceptual distinctions, measurement challenges, and research agenda. Adm Policy Ment Health 2011;38(2):65–76.
161. Lewis CC, Fischer S, Weiner BJ, et al. Outcomes for implementation science: an enhanced systematic review of instruments using evidence-based rating criteria. Implement Sci 2015;10:155.
162. Jungnick S, Hobmaier B, Mautner L, et al. Detection of the new SARS-CoV-2 variants of concern B.1.1.7 and B.1.351 in five SARS-CoV-2 rapid antigen tests (RATs), Germany, March 2021. Euro Surveill 2021;26(16):2100413.

Alternative Methods to Detect Severe Acute Respiratory Syndrome Coronavirus 2 Antibodies

Rashmi Patel, MBBS, MS[a], Siddharth Khare, PhD[a],
Vinay S. Mahajan, MBBS, PhD[b,c],*

KEYWORDS

- Serology • Immunoassay • ELISA • SARS-CoV-2 • Electrochemical detection
- Luminescence • Neutralization assay

KEY POINTS

- Lateral flow assays (LFA) and enzyme-linked immunosorbent assays (ELISA) are the cornerstones of SARS-CoV-2 serologic diagnosis.
- A comprehensive serologic analysis involves determining the response to multiple viral antigens, and antibody characteristics, such as isotype and neutralization potential.
- Technical advances in photonics, electrochemistry, protein design, luminescence probes, and nanotechnology have been applied to serologic diagnostics of SARS-CoV-2; these assays are in varying stages of development.
- Serologic assays for SARS-CoV-2, and especially neutralization assays, need to keep up with the emergence of viral variants, necessitating a high degree of vigilance among laboratory practitioners.

INTRODUCTION

The SARS-CoV-2 pandemic resulted in an intense demand for serologic diagnostics, leading to the development of hundreds of assays across the world, especially lateral flow assays (LFAs). The COVID-19 test directory on the FindDx Web site includes an exhaustive catalog of these assays.[1] By June 2021, the US Food Drug Administration (FDA) had issued Emergency Use Authorizations (EUA) for 80 serologic tests for SARS-CoV-2.[2] These range from rapid qualitative LFAs to semiquantitative enzyme-linked immunosorbent assays (ELISAs) and include assays that are performed on fully

[a] Micelio Labs, 58, 15th Cross Road, 2nd Phase, J P Nagar, Bengaluru 560078, India; [b] Ragon Institute of MGH, MIT and Harvard, 400 Technology Square, Cambridge, MA 02139, USA; [c] Department of Pathology, Brigham and Women's Hospital, 75 Francis St, Boston, MA 02215, USA
* Corresponding author. Ragon Institute of MGH, MIT and Harvard400 Technology Square, Cambridge, MA 02139, USA.
E-mail address: vinay.mahajan@mgh.harvard.edu

Clin Lab Med 42 (2022) 57–73
https://doi.org/10.1016/j.cll.2021.10.007
0272-2712/22/© 2021 Elsevier Inc. All rights reserved.

labmed.theclinics.com

automated laboratory analyzers. In most COVID-infected patients, antibodies are observed approximately 1 to 2 weeks following symptom onset or polymerase chain reaction positivity in symptomatic or asymptomatic individuals, respectively.[3,4] The observed timing of seroconversion also depends on the sensitivity of the assay. Seroconversion may be picked up as early as the day of the first positive nucleic acid test after symptom onset with ultrasensitive single-molecule approaches (Simoa, Quanterix Technologies, Billerica, MA).[5] Unlike typical seroconversion profiles in other infectious contexts, near-simultaneous production of IgM, IgG, and IgA has been observed in patients with confirmed SARS-CoV-2.[6,7] Although IgM titers may disappear within a month, IgG titers are detectable for much longer but also exhibit a gradual decline in the months following infection.[8–10] Higher antibody titers are seen following symptomatic or severe disease.[11]

The serologic assays that have been developed have focused on the structural proteins of the virus, that is, spike and nucleocapsid. Spike is a transmembrane glycoprotein comprising two parts, S1 and S2. The binding of the SARS-CoV-2 spike to its receptor, angiotensin-converting enzyme 2 (ACE2), is mediated by S1. S2 mediates fusion of the viral envelope to the cell membrane and cell entry during infection. The S1 receptor binding domain (RBD) binds ACE2 and is highly immunogenic. The spike protein contains sequences unique to SARS-CoV-2 and shared with other betacoronaviruses. Thus, assessing the serologic response to antigens from other human coronaviruses can help exclude cross-reactive responses. Determining the antibody isotype (eg, IgM, IgG, or IgA) may provide additional information for determining immune status. Unlike natural infection, most vaccines induce antispike but not antinucleocapsid responses and IgG rather than IgA. These characteristics may help distinguish between vaccine-induced responses and natural infection. Vaccines are designed to elicit antibodies against the S1 RBD because antibodies to this region can neutralize the virus. Thus, in addition to antibody specificity, a complete serologic characterization involves determining the isotype and neutralization potential.

There is a great interest in using serologic parameters to determine infection risk, vaccine efficacy, or vaccine prioritization. However, serologic assays do not detect the presence of memory B or T cells, and it is possible that memory lymphocytes may offer some immunity in subjects with declining antibody titers.[12] The relationship between seropositivity or neutralization titers and protection remains unknown and is being evaluated in clinical and epidemiologic studies. Given the rise of SARS-CoV-2 variants and the variable magnitude of serologic responses among convalescent individuals, the use of serology as a surrogate for protection is likely to remain a controversial and changing landscape. Because of the previously mentioned uncertainties, the Centers for Disease Control and Prevention and FDA have advised against the use of serologic assays for assessing protection, and interpretive guidance is imperative while reporting a serologic test result.[13] Given their utility in a point-of-care setting, LFAs for antibodies have been widely used in population serosurveys to estimate exposure rates and guide public health policy. Seroconversion indicates prior exposure but not active infection, and LFAs that detect viral antigens rather than antibodies should be used to determine infectious risk.[14]

Although manufacturers monitor performance using traceability to recognized standards, independent monitoring of assay performance by clinical laboratories was especially vital in ensuring that these assays were effectively used during a time that witnessed widespread supply chain disruptions with the potential to impact assay manufacturing and distribution. Indeed, when concerns were raised about the reliability of certain LFAs, the EUA for some assays were revoked by the FDA. Independent vigilance of serologic assays by clinical laboratory practitioners continues to be important because the antigen formulation used in the serologic tests has remained unchanged despite the emergence of SARS-CoV-2 variants. In particular, the interpretation of neutralization assays may be significantly impacted by SARS-CoV-2 variants. Variants that may have an enhanced capacity to evade neutralizing antibodies are referred to as variants of concern.[15] Such variants are likely to keep emerging as the virus continues to evolve in the face of immune pressure when herd immunity builds up in a population.[16] Although the FDA has issued an EUA for one ELISA-based qualitative neutralization assay (cPass, GenScript, Piscataway, NJ), it is only intended to assess recent infection and its clinical applicability to determine the degree of immunity is not known. Most neutralization assays are high-complexity tests and are performed by specialized laboratories. They have primarily been used by vaccine developers and need nuanced interpretation in the light of concerns about variants of concern. The continued emergence of variants raises concerns about the need to update the assays to assess neutralization capacity against emerging variants. We have described neutralization assays in detail in a separate section.

There is a need for the development of reliable and clinically scalable multiplexed serologic assays, suitable for point-of-care use. Some of these challenges may be addressed by adopting emerging alternate technologies. This article highlights a few novel and alternative approaches that rely on electrochemical analysis, luminescent signals, or label-free optical detection. Ultrasensitive and quantitative approaches, such as Simoa (Quanterix Technologies), have now entered the market, which has opened a range of novel possibilities in serologic diagnostics, but these instruments are not widely available. However, they have also been used as a quantitative reference method to compare the performance of other serologic assays across a broad range of antibody dilutions.[17] We emphasize that many of the approaches described in this article are still in development and are yet to receive regulatory clearance. This article is also not meant to be an exhaustive review of alternative approaches to serology; it is divided into sections based on the physical principle used for assay signal generation.

GENERAL PRINCIPLES OF A SEROLOGIC ASSAY

Broadly, a serologic assay involves a mechanism for signal generation, signal amplification, and signal detection (**Fig. 1**). If the unbound label can generate a signal on

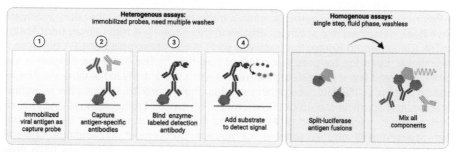

Fig. 1. General principles of an immunoassay. A heterogeneous immunoassay for antigen-specific antibodies relies on immobilized antigen as a capture probe and often uses enzyme labels for signal amplification; it requires stepwise reagent addition with multiple washes. A homogeneous immunoassay is washless and generates a signal only in the presence of the target analyte. An assay devised using antigens fused to split-luciferase domains is shown as an example.

its own, it needs to be separated by washing before measurement. Such an assay is called "heterogeneous." If the label generates a signal only in presence of the analyte, the immunoassay can be performed in a washless or "homogeneous" format. If the signal can be quantitatively measured across a sufficiently wide dynamic range, the assay can be calibrated with a range of accepted standards to generate a quantitative result. Some approaches are based on label-free or direct measurement of the physical or chemical changes induced by antibody binding, and do not require the use of a labeled secondary antibody as a detection probe.

After incubation of patient serum with the specimen and removal of unbound antibodies, the antigen-bound antibodies are measured using a labeled detection probe, such as anti-IgG or anti-IgM. Such a setup is called a sandwich immunoassay (see **Fig. 1**). When the detection probe is labeled with an enzyme to amplify a signal-generating chemical reaction, it is called a sandwich ELISA. ELISAs are typically coupled to an optical signal. Test sensitivity and specificity are established based on comparison against established positive and negative samples based on polymerase chain reaction positivity. Prepandemic specimens have been used as negative control subjects. For all assays that were issued an EUA, the FDA has published estimates of sensitivity and specificity on its Web site.[18] However, these numbers are estimates with 95% confidence intervals and positive and negative predictive values depend on the prevalence. The kinetics of seroconversion and the potential loss of titers on convalescence should be considered when interpreting negative results.

The design of each assay step influences the overall signal-to-noise ratio and consequently the sensitivity and specificity of the test. SARS-CoV-2 antigens, typically spike or nucleocapsid proteins, are used as capture probes for antibodies. Some assays include other human coronaviral antigens as specificity controls. Blocking of nonspecific binding is especially important for minimizing the background signal in assays where antibodies bound to an antigen-coated surface are measured. The choice and source of the antigens may also influence their antigenicity and contribute to differences in performance between assays that detect the same antigen. For instance, the spike protein may be used as a capture probe in its full-length form, or just the S1 domain or RBD alone. However, the full-length spike protein is less stable than the S1 domain or RBD. The approach used for surface coupling may also impact antigenic stability and access to antigenic epitopes.[19] The antigens need to be stabilized especially for use in a point-of-care setting without refrigerated storage. Antigenicity is also influenced by glycosylation, and thus fully glycosylated antigens expressed in a mammalian host are likely to best capture the full breadth of the serologic response.

Point-of-care LFAs and serologic assays performed on central laboratory analyzers have been described in concurrent articles in this issue. The rapid assay from Nano-EnTek (Seoul, South Korea) that received an FDA EUA resembles an LFA but uses a microfluidic cartridge for precise control of fluid flow.[20] The fluorescent signal in the cartridge is read using a dedicated instrument with connectivity to the laboratory information system. ELISA kits, which can yield quantitative results, are typically manufactured as microparticle-based or 96-well microtiter-based immunoassays and require manual setup, washing, and a plate reader. This involves significant infrastructure and operator skill and is suitable for medium throughput applications. Several COVID-19 serologic assays for automated central laboratory analyzers have now become available and should be considered for high-throughput operations. In this article, we have focused on serologic assays that use alternate or unconventional detection methodologies. These assays may help bridge the gap between LFAs and central laboratory analyzers in terms of assay performance and throughput. Although many of the approaches described in this article are proof-of-principle demonstrations and are yet to be commercialized or implemented in a clinical setting, a few have received an FDA EUA. The assays from Genaltye (San Diego, CA; Maverick Multi-Antigen Serology Panel) and Genscript (cPass) are two such examples and are among those described in this article.[21,22] Among other serologic assays that have received an EUA and rely on an unconventional detection approach, the assays from MosaicQ (Quotient Diagnostics Ltd, United Kingdom) and Luminex (Austin, TX) are noteworthy; they are solid-phase ELISAs that use light scattering or fluorescence properties of nanoparticles for sensitive or multiplexed detection.[23,24] Both platforms can be combined with antigen tests. However, a specialized instrument is required for analysis.

ELECTROCHEMICAL IMMUNOASSAYS

This approach relies on the functionalization of the surface of a working electrode in an electrochemical cell with desired antigens.[25] Antibody binding to the electrode surface results in quantitative changes in electrical properties, such as impedance, which is measured in a label-free and washless setup (**Fig. 2**). Alternatively, antibody binding is coupled to a reduction-oxidation (redox) reaction, such as one catalyzed by the widely used ELISA label, horseradish peroxidase (HRP), and the generated current is measured in a low-cost setup (see **Fig. 2**). A few such assays have been implemented in the context of COVID-19 serology as a proof-of-concept and are listed next.

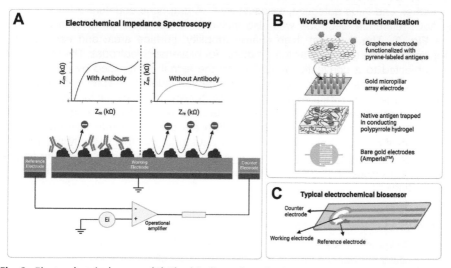

Fig. 2. Electrochemical assays. (*A*) The binding of antibodies to antigens coated on the surface of a working electrode impedes electron transport, and results in a quantitative change in impedance. This is measured using various electrochemical impedance spectroscopy techniques. For instance, as illustrated using Nyquist plots, the frequency dependence of the impedance is influenced by a change in the surface properties of the electrode when it is bound by an antibody. (*B*) Two approaches to functionalize a working electrode are shown. A graphene electrode is functionalized with noncovalently stacked pyrene-labeled antigens; such a graphene layer can also be coated on gold electrodes. Electrodes used in the Amperial platform are functionalized with native antigens entrapped in a conducting polypyrrole hydrogel using in situ electropolymerization. (*C*) A typical electrochemical electrode design comprising a working electrode, a counterelectrode, and a reference electrode.

Amperometric Enzyme-Linked Immunosorbent Assay in Microtiter Plates

The Amperial assay platform (Liquid Diagnostics, San Clemente, CA) is designed to implement an ELISA assay with an electrochemical readout.[26] It uses microtiter plates fabricated with gold electrodes at the bottom of each well. First, the surface of the electrode is functionalized with the target antigen by electropolymerizing a pyrrole solution containing native antigens. This entraps antigens in a native state on the surface of the electrode within a conductive polypyrrole hydrogel. Next a sandwich ELISA is performed with an HRP-labeled secondary antibody for detection (see **Fig. 2**). On addition of a redox substrate and the application of a voltage, the peroxidase reaction produces an electric current that serves as a quantitative assay readout. A sensitivity greater than 88% and specificity greater than 99.85% was observed with S1 antigen. The immobilization of native antigen in an electropolymerized polypyrrole hydrogel preserves its antigenicity and offers the flexibility to test various types of antigens. The assay is quantitative, and the current in nanoamperes is read for the whole plate within 3 minutes. However, it is a conventional heterogeneous sandwich immunoassay involving multiple wash steps.

Multiplexed Miniaturized Amperometric Enzyme-Linked Immunosorbent Assay

A scalable low-cost laser-engraving technique was used to fabricate a miniaturized arrangement of disposable printed graphene electrodes individually functionalized with S1 domain, nucleocapsid antigen, C-reactive protein, and an antinucleocapsid antibody for simultaneously assessing the serologic response, an inflammatory biomarker, and virus detection, respectively.[27] A graphene counterelectrode and an Ag/AgCl reference electrode was also included to complete the biosensor circuit (see **Fig. 2**). The low cost, high charge mobility, surface area, and ease of bioconjugation make graphene an ideal material for biosensor electrodes. The biosensors are subjected to a conventional ELISA and the signal is amplified by HRP-labeled detection antibodies that produce an amperometric readout in the presence of a redox substrate. The device is linked to a compact battery-powered circuit that transmits the signal to a cellphone via Bluetooth. Analytical sensitivity of 1 pm was achieved with only 10 minutes of specimen incubation. The electrode was manually rinsed with wash buffers and incubated with the redox substrate, but this is easily automated. Comparable sensitivity was seen with saliva and serum. The study showed the potential of this approach in a quantitative, multiplexed assay that is suitable for point-of-care settings.[26]

Repurposed Cellular Impedance Monitoring Platform

The xCELLigence system (Agilent, Santa Clara, CA) is an instrument designed to detect cellular impedance for real-time monitoring of cell cultures with label-free measurement of cellular function, such as cell growth, shape, or toxicity. The cells are grown and monitored in specially fabricated plates with an electrode at the base of each well. If, however, the same multiwell cell culture plates are used to perform an ELISA with coated antigens, the change in impedance as a result of antibody binding is measured in a washless format.[28] This was tested with S1 and RBD antigens. Antibody binding led to a sharp increase in impedance followed by a gradual decay over several minutes. Antibody binding is rapidly detected in a washless format, within minutes. This was an experimental demonstration of electrochemical measurement of SARS-CoV-2 serology by repurposing a device already in use in some research laboratories.

Label-Free Electrochemical Immunoassay Using a Gold Micropillar Array Electrode

A three-dimensional gold microelectrode array was fabricated and decorated with reduced graphene oxide, and then conjugated to the SARS-CoV-2 spike protein; the three-dimensional geometry of the electrode results in a stronger current and also permits immobilization of the antigen at a higher density, resulting in greater antibody capture.[29] S1 and RBD were tested and yielded a quantitative measurement range of 1 pm to 10 nM. A change in impedance was detected within 3 seconds of incubation. The signal is saturated over 10-nM concentration when all available binding sites on the sensor surface are occupied by the specific antibodies. A low-cost coin-sized portable electrochemical impedance spectroscopy analyzer (Sensit, PalmSens, Houten, the Netherlands) connected to a smartphone was used for measurements. This approach offers label-free detection with a few microliters of blood. The biosensor is regenerated and reused after removing the bound antibodies with pH 2.5 formic acid. The sensor has a high regeneration capability with a good signal output even after nine regeneration cycles. The electrodes require specialized techniques for fabrication, but the assay characteristics are suitable for point-of-care use.

A Paper-Based Electrochemical Biosensor

A simple label-free rapid paper-based electrochemical serology sensor was implemented with RBD antigen immobilized on printed graphene electrodes in a vertical flow assay format.[30] Antibody binding was detected using an electrochemical spectroscopy technique called square wave voltammetry using a portable PalmSens analyzer. In this technique, the signal-to-noise ratio increases by the square root of the scan rate. The improved signal is a function of the time between pulse application and the current measurement, and the change in the faradaic current is measured as peaks on the voltammogram. The test was performed with patient sera and compared with a homemade colorimetric LFA device, prepared using the same batch of RBD. It exhibited better sensitivity for detection of IgM compared with IgG because of its larger size. It is a low-cost, rapid qualitative test suitable for point-of-care use with greater sensitivity compared with conventional LFAs, but requires an electrochemical impedance spectroscopy analyzer for readout. Being a label-free approach, unlike conventional immunosandwich LFAs, it is not impacted by the risk of false-negatives because of the high-dose "hook effect" or prozone phenomenon.

BIOLUMINESCENT LABELS

Luminescent labels, which catalyze a light-emitting chemical reaction, are widely used for sensitive detection using ELISAs. Unlike colorimetric or fluorescence detection, a light source or excitation is not required, and this approach offers greater sensitivity, lower background, and a wide dynamic range using inexpensive instrumentation. The collected photons are amplified into a current signal that is reported as relative light units. Several luminescent substrates for the widely used immunoperoxidase or alkaline phosphatase labels have been developed and they form the basis of most modern ELISAs. Bioluminescence refers to analogous reactions observed in living organisms that are catalyzed by specialized enzymes called luciferases acting on substrates called luciferins. The luciferase-luciferin systems have been adapted to build highly sensitive immunoassays. These assays have been implemented in a fluid-phase ELISA and homogeneous washless formats using antigen-luciferase fusion proteins, split luciferases, or designer proteins. Their broad dynamic range allows measurement across decades of concentration

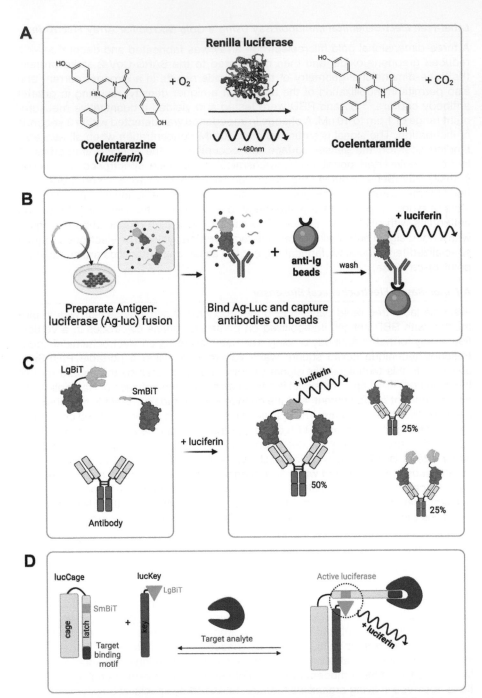

Fig. 3. Bioluminescence assays. (*A*) Luciferase is an enzyme that catalyzes a bioluminescent reaction by oxidizing a luciferin substrate. Luciferase systems that are well-characterized are widely used in bioassays (Renilla luciferase and coelenterazine substrate are shown). (*B*) LIPS. Crude lysate bearing recombinant antigen-luciferase fusion protein is incubated with serum and antibodies are pulled down with anti-Ig beads. Antigen-specific antibodies

without the need for sample dilutions. The reagent systems for luminescent reactions are more complex than those used for spectrophotometric and fluorometric analyses and require more careful control and low temperature storage. Furthermore, luminescence measurements must follow the kinetics of the reaction. Although rapid luciferin oxidation can produce a bright signal, signal detection may need to be timed with the injection of the luciferin substrate.

Luciferase Immunoprecipitation Assay

Luciferase immunoprecipitation (LIPS) assays are heterogeneous liquid-phase immunoassays (**Fig. 3**A and **3**B).[31,32] Unlike ELISA, which is typically a solid-phase assay, antibody-antigen binding takes place in the fluid phase in an LIPS assay, thus better maintaining the native antigen conformation. Luciferase-labeled antigens are expressed as recombinant fusion proteins. The ability to use crude cell lysates of mammalian cells transfected with an antigen-luciferase fusion protein expression vector without further purification greatly simplifies assay development. This was particularly helpful for rapid development of these assays in the early days of the pandemic when antigens were not readily available. It also allows the rapid development of serologic tests for antigens from variants of concern without the need for purified antigens. A single preparation of crude lysates containing antigen-luciferase fusion protein can be used for thousands of assays. However, various configurations of antigen-luciferase fusions need to be tested and optimized during assay development. Luminescence is measured on addition of the luciferase substrate using a microplate reader, yielding a quantitative result with high analytical sensitivity and a wide dynamic range without the need for sample dilution. LIPS assays have been implemented using luciferase fused to nucleocapsid and spike proteins.[31] For IgG against nucleocapsid, the sensitivity and specificity were 100% at 14 days after the onset of symptoms (n = 35). For IgG against spike, sensitivity of 94% and specificity of 100% was observed.

Engineering Luminescent Biosensors for Point-of-Care SARS-CoV-2 Antibody Detection

This approach uses rationally designed antibody biosensors based on split nanoluciferase fragments (SmBiT and LgBiT) fused to SARS-CoV-2 antigens (**Fig. 3**C).[33] Because an antibody has two fragment antigen-binding (Fab) arms, incubating the specimen with a 1:1 mix of SmBiT and LgBiT biosensors results in half of the antiviral antibodies binding LgBiT with one Fab arm and SmBiT with the other Fab arm. If the antigen binding orientation is such that it brings the LgBiT and

---

are measured using a luciferase signal. (*C*) Split nanoluciferase fragments (large BiT [LgBit] and small BiT [SmBiT]) are fused to RBD. An active nanoluciferase is assembled on bivalent antibody binding, which is sensitively detected with a luciferase substrate in a homogeneous assay format. (*D*) A de novo designed lucCage:lucKey protein biosensor. The lucCage protein is built with a cage domain and a latch domain, which contains a target-binding motif and a split luciferase fragment (SmBit). The lucKey contains a key peptide that binds the lucCage cage domain and the complementary split luciferase fragment (LgBit). Binding of the analyte to the lucCage latch stabilizes the open conformation of lucCage, interaction with the lucKey, and assembly of an intact luciferase. The thermodynamics of the system are designed such that the intact luciferase is reconstituted only in the presence of the target analyte.

SmBiT fragments into close proximity, it results in the reconstitution of an intact, enzymatically active nanoluciferase enzyme. This is used for luminescence-based detection of antigen-specific antibodies in a homogeneous assay format. Sensors for RBD and nucleocapsid were designed using this approach and shown to require less than 30 minutes to result, suitable for point-of-care applications.[33] It is sensitive enough for testing serum or plasma (>99% sensitivity) and to a lesser extent saliva (79% sensitive).

De Novo Designed Protein Biosensor with Miniprotein Sensing Domains

Although once considered impossible, the explosion in the knowledge of protein structure and folding has led to the realization of de novo designed proteins.[34] One such rationally designed modular protein biosensor (lucCage and lucKey) was built such that antibody binding to the biosensor is thermodynamically coupled to switching from a closed dark state and an open luminescent state (**Fig. 3**D).[35] This biosensor is used in a homogeneous assay format and was built with RBD as the antigen. Antibodies against RBD could be detected at a sensitivity of 15 pm with a signal over background of more than 50-fold. The lucCage biosensor is based on thermodynamic coupling between defined closed and open states of the system; thus, its sensitivity depends on the free energy change on the binding of the sensing domain to the target but not the specific binding geometry. This enables the incorporation of various binding modalities, including small peptides, globular miniproteins, antibody epitopes, and de novo designed binders, to generate sensitive sensors for a wide range of protein targets with little or no optimization. For point-of-care applications, the system has the advantages of being homogeneous, no-wash, and gives a nearly instantaneous readout; the quantification of luminescence is carried out with inexpensive and accessible devices, such as a cell phone camera. The ability to modularly design sensors with identical readouts for diverse antigens could enable multiplexed serologic assays using an array of different sensors. However, there is considerable variation between different sensors in the level of activation at saturating target concentrations.

LABEL-FREE OPTICAL APPROACHES

Nanoscale changes resulting from the binding of a protein to an optical surface is amplified and detected by specialized optical techniques or devices, such as surface plasmon resonance, biolayer interferometry, optical cavities, or resonators.[36,37] They have been commercialized into benchtop instruments and we highlight two approaches that have been applied to serologic diagnosis of SARS-CoV-2. Semiconductor-based photonic technologies are rapidly evolving, and such devices may soon become more commonplace.

Biolayer Interferometry

Biolayer interferometry is used to measure the binding of a protein in solution to an immobilized ligand on a biosensor tip (**Fig. 4**A). The biolayer interferometry instrument (Octet, Sartorius, Göttingen, Germany) is increasingly used in the research and biotechnology space. Protein binding produces an increase in optical thickness at the biosensor tip, altering the interference pattern of reflected light. This approach was used to build a proof-of-concept assay for the rapid and semiquantitative measurement of SARS-CoV-2 antibodies in saliva and plasma and is called biolayer interferometry immunosorbent assay.[36] Rapid real-time and quantitative antibody binding data are obtained in less than 20 minutes in a washless and

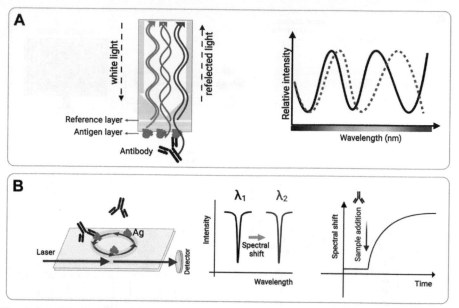

Fig. 4. Label-free optics. (*A*) Biolayer interferometry relies on measuring the interference pattern of white light reflected from an internal reference layer and the biosensor tip coated with antigen. Binding of antibodies to the test surface can shift the optical path by a few nanometers and this is detected by analyzing the interference pattern. This approach allows real-time monitoring of protein binding and dissociation and is compatible with crude samples because the surrounding medium does not influence these measurements. (*B*) An optical ring biosensor is an optical cavity that is functionalized with antigen and coupled to a tunable laser. A dip in the signal intensity of a tunable laser is used to determine the resonant wavelength of the optical ring. Binding of an analyte results in a shift in the resonant wavelength, which can be monitored in real time.

label-free fashion. Various sample types, such as saliva and serum, are tested on the same platform. The sensitivity and specificity were not assessed with clinical specimens.

Optical Ring Resonators

The diagnostic applications of optical ring resonators have been commercialized by Genalyte. An optical ring resonator is a type of optical wave-guide-based biosensor that traps light passing along an adjacent linear waveguide at its resonance frequency (**Fig. 4**B).[37] The light makes multiple passes in the resonator allowing for larger effective interaction length (several centimeters) and improving the sensitivity of detection. This also significantly reduces the physical size of the sensor. Antibody binding to antigen coated on the ring resonator results in a detectable shift in its resonant frequency proportional to the mass of bound biomolecules. Primary and secondary antibodies are flowed over the biosensor and detected in real-time with a tunable laser. The assay protocols take less than 15 minutes and are run on an automated platform (Maverick, Genalyte), which supports a large number of immunoassays in addition to Sars-CoV-2 serology.[38] A SARS-CoV-2 Multi-Antigen Serology Panel was developed by Genalyte on this platform and was issued an EUA by the FDA. The assay performance is similar to other fully automated platforms. It includes an array of antigens, including spike proteins from other human coronaviruses as specificity controls.[21,39]

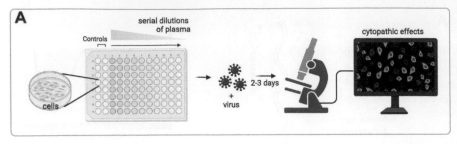

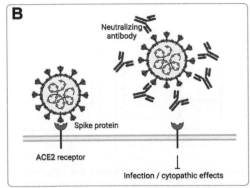

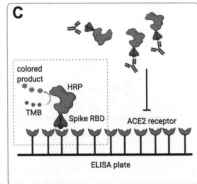

Fig. 5. Neutralization assays. (*A*) A neutralization assay is typically set up using cells cultured in a multiwell plate. The ability of serial dilutions of test serum to interfere with virus-induced cytopathic effects using a predetermined dose of infectious virus is measured. (*B*) Neutralization assay detects the presence of antibodies, which can prevent the infection or cell entry of infectious SARS-CoV-2. Alternatively, reporter viruses pseudotyped with the SARS-CoV-2 spike protein and that rely on spike protein for cell entry are used at a lower biosafety level. (*C*) Surrogate neutralization assay relies on measuring the ability of the specimen to interfere with the binding of surface-bound ACE2 receptor with spike protein or RBD in a competitive ELISA. (TMB - 3,3',5,5'-Tetramethylbenzidine)

NEUTRALIZATION ASSAYS

A virus neutralization test (VNT) is a serologic test used to quantify the subset of antibodies that can prevent viral infection (**Fig. 5**). Such antibodies are called neutralizing antibodies, and in the case of SARS-CoV-2 infection or vaccination, they interfere with binding to its cellular receptor ACE2 and inhibit viral entry. Conventional VNTs are used alongside an infectivity assay (eg, plaque assay) to assess the ability of antibodies to inhibit viral replication or neutralize viral infection, which takes 2 to 4 days to complete. Surrogate VNTs that measure the ability of antibodies to block the interaction between the spike and ACE2 proteins have also been devised. Seropositivity against spike protein measured by commercial assays does correlate with neutralization activity.[40,41] The specimens that did not correlate with neutralization activity also exhibited greater discordance among serologic assays from different manufacturers, suggesting that a neutralization assay could also be used for improving the specificity of a conventional serologic assay because other common human betacoronaviruses do not use ACE2 as a receptor. Because of the dimeric nature of secreted IgA in saliva, it has been shown to be 15 times more potent at neutralization than its monomeric form in plasma.[42] This highlights the potential value of measuring isotype-specific neutralization, which is typically not done. Neutralization assays have primarily been used in research, epidemiologic studies, or vaccine development; their role in routine clinical diagnostics is yet to be defined.

Cellular Virus Neutralization Assays

Conventional VNTs measure the infection of a susceptible cell line with a defined amount of a specific replication competent SARS-CoV-2 strain in the presence of varying dilutions of the plasma. Multiple viral strains may be used to assess neutralization breadth. The resulting infectious virions are quantified using a plaque assay that can take an additional 2 to 4 days. Alternatively, cytopathic effects are observed and the estimated dilution at which 50% of the wells show a cytopathic effects is reported as tissue-culture infectious dose (TCID50). The neutralizing titer is reported as the dilution required to produce a 50% reduction in infectious virions (PRNT50). Although this is the gold standard approach, it is a labor-intensive protocol that takes several days and needs to be performed in specialized biosafety facilities, because SARS-CoV-2 culture requires a higher biosafety level (BSL3). Recently, a high throughput label-free optical approach called laser force cytology that examines cellular deformability using optical tweezers in a microfluidic channel (Radiance, LumaCyte, Charlottesville, VA) has been adapted to count virally infected cells to automate the readout of VNTs.[43] To overcome the BSL3 requirements, pseudotyped retroviruses or replication-defective VSV particles have been engineered that use the SARS-CoV-2 spike for cell entry. The pseudotyped viruses are used in neutralization assays in a conventional BSL2 laboratory and show good agreement with assays using replication-competent SARS-CoV-2.[44] Furthermore, pseudotyped viruses have also been engineered to express a fluorescent or luciferase reporter for ease of measurement and scalability in a clinical setting. The IMMUNOCOV assay that uses pseudotyped VSV-G engineered with a luciferase reporter is commercially available; sufficient virus reagent has been banked to test 5 million clinical samples.[45] VNTs based on surrogate engineered viruses are readily adapted to study neutralization of variants by incorporating spike mutations from variants of interest.

Surrogate Virus Neutralization Assays

Surrogate VNTs that assess the ability of antiviral antibodies to inhibit the interaction between the viral receptor (ACE2) and the spike protein have been devised (see **Fig. 5C**). Surrogate VNT assays may miss neutralizing antibodies that interfere with downstream steps of cell entry following ACE2 receptor binding involving membrane fusion and cell entry. Thus, the full spectrum of neutralizing capacity is most reliably measured using neutralization assays that rely on a live virus. ELISA-format surrogate VNTs require the lowest biosafety level and yield a result within hours but may miss samples with lower neutralizing capacity. Once such assay, cPass (GenScript), has received an FDA EUA.[22] Updated ELISA assays that assess the neutralization of emerging variants are under development (Axim Biotechnologies, San Diego, CA). Surrogate VNTs can also be implemented using other rapid approaches including LFAs (eg, NeuCOVIX, Axim Biotechnologies).

FUTURE DIRECTIONS

We have highlighted selected alternative approaches to the serologic diagnosis of SARS-CoV-2. A broad variety of biosensors harnessing nanoscale phenomena, nanopore physics, oligonucleotide chemistry, or next-generation sequencing have been proposed in the literature, some of which have been applied to SARS-CoV-2 serology.[46–48] Nanomaterial phenomena have also been exploited to enhance the performance of LFAs.[49] Although such approaches can be applied toward improving the characterization of the antibody response, a serologic assay does not provide complete information about humoral immunity. For instance, persistent antigen-specific memory B cells are not directly assessed by serologic tests. Furthermore, the cellular immune response consisting of $CD4^+$ and $CD8^+$ T cells is integral to the immune response, and a comprehensive assessment may be required to better assess infection risk. The T-Detect COVID test (Adaptive Biotechnologies, Seattle WA) based on the analysis of the T-cell repertoire by next-generation sequencing is a step in this direction.[50] Although the bulk of the serologic diagnostics have focused on blood specimens, it has been shown that the antibodies to SARS-CoV-2 found in the saliva do correlate well with levels in the blood.[51] Serologic monitoring of saliva may offer a noninvasive alternative to monitor seropositivity at a population scale.[52] Rapid advances have been made in SARS-CoV-2 serology, but concomitant measurement of cellular immunity is critical in obtaining a comprehensive picture of immunity in the context of natural infection, vaccine-induced protection, or population surveys of immunity. Use of novel or alternate technologies is required to develop assays for clinically scalable and multiplexed assessment of immune function in COVID-19.

CLINICS CARE POINTS

- The clinical utility of serological assays is currently limited in the context of SARS-CoV-2, but they have been most impactful in seroprevalence studies. Further studies are needed to determine the correlates of protection.
- The adoption of emerging technologies for comprehensive assessment of the immune response including assessment of the T cell response will be needed to provide better correlates of immunity and protection.

ACKNOWLEDGMENTS

All figures were created with BioRender.com

DISCLOSURE

R. Patel and S. Khare are affiliated with Micelio Labs, India, a technology incubator focused on artificial intelligence, health care, and diagnostics.

REFERENCES

1. FindDx test directory. Available at: https://www.finddx.org/test-directory/. Accessed May 23, 2021.
2. EUAs: serology and other adaptive immune response tests for SARS-CoV-2. Available at: https://www.fda.gov/medical-devices/coronavirus-disease-2019-covid-19-emergency-use-authorizations-medical-devices/in-vitro-diagnostics-euas-serology-and-other-adaptive-immune-response-tests-sars-cov-2#individual-serological. Accessed June 17, 2021.
3. Sethuraman N, Jeremiah SS, Ryo A. Interpreting diagnostic tests for SARS-CoV-2. JAMA 2020;323(22):2249–51.
4. Maine GN, Lao KM, Krishnan SM, et al. Longitudinal characterization of the IgM and IgG humoral response in symptomatic COVID-19 patients using the Abbott Architect. J Clin Virol 2020;133:104663.

5. Norman M, Gilboa T, Ogata AF, et al. Ultrasensitive high-resolution profiling of early seroconversion in patients with COVID-19. Nat Biomed Eng 2020;4(12): 1180–7.

6. Orner EP, Rodgers MA, Hock K, et al. Comparison of SARS-CoV-2 IgM and IgG seroconversion profiles among hospitalized patients in two US cities. Diagn Microbiol Infect Dis 2021;99(4):115300.

7. Sterlin D, Mathian A, Miyara M, et al. IgA dominates the early neutralizing antibody response to SARS-CoV-2 n.d. Sci Transl Med 2021. https://doi.org/10. 1101/2020.06.10.20126532.

8. Van Elslande J, Oyaert M, Ailliet S, et al. Longitudinal follow-up of IgG antinucleocapsid antibodies in SARS-CoV-2 infected patients up to eight months after infection. J Clin Virol 2021;136:104765.

9. Lumley SF, Wei J, O'Donnell D, et al. The duration, dynamics and determinants of SARS-CoV-2 antibody responses in individual healthcare workers. Clin Infect Dis 2021. https://doi.org/10.1093/cid/ciab004.

10. Crawford KHD, Dingens AS, Eguia R, et al. Dynamics of neutralizing antibody titers in the months after SARS-CoV-2 infection. J Infect Dis 2020. https://doi.org/ 10.1093/infdis/jiaa618.

11. Röltgen K, Powell AE, Wirz OF, et al. Defining the features and duration of antibody responses to SARS-CoV-2 infection associated with disease severity and outcome. Sci Immunol 2020;5(54). https://doi.org/10.1126/sciimmunol.abe0240.

12. Turner JS, Kim W, Kalaidina E, et al. SARS-CoV-2 infection induces long-lived bone marrow plasma cells in humans. Nature 2021. https://doi.org/10.1038/ s41586-021-03647-4.

13. Bermingham WH, Wilding T, Beck S, et al. SARS-CoV-2 serology: test, test, test, but interpret with caution. Clin Med 2020;20(4):365–8.

14. Mina MJ, Parker R, Larremore DB. Rethinking Covid-19 test sensitivity: a strategy for containment. N Engl J Med 2020;383(22):e120.

15. Geers D, Shamier MC, Bogers S, et al. SARS-CoV-2 variants of concern partially escape humoral but not T-cell responses in COVID-19 convalescent donors and vaccinees. Sci Immunol 2021;6(59). https://doi.org/10.1126/sciimmunol.abj1750.

16. Harvey WT, Carabelli AM, Jackson B, et al. SARS-CoV-2 variants, spike mutations and immune escape. Nat Rev Microbiol 2021;19(7):409–24.

17. Trombetta BA, Kandigian SE, Kitchen RR, et al. Evaluation of serological lateral flow assays for severe acute respiratory syndrome coronavirus-2. BMC Infect Dis 2021;21(1):1–14.

18. EUA authorized serology test performance. Available at: https://www.fda.gov/ medical-devices/coronavirus-disease-2019-covid-19-emergency-use-authorizations-medical-devices/eua-authorized-serology-test-performance. Accessed June 21, 2021.

19. Liu G, Rusling JF. COVID-19 antibody tests and their limitations. ACS Sens 2021; 6(3):593–612.

20. Orsi A, Pennati BM, Bruzzone B, et al. On-field evaluation of a ultra-rapid fluorescence immunoassay as a frontline test for SARS-CoV-2 diagnostic. J Virol Methods 2021;295:114201.

21. Ikegami S, Benirschke RC, Fakhrai-Rad H, et al. Target specific serologic analysis of COVID-19 convalescent plasma. PLoS One 2021;16(4):e0249938.

22. Murray MJ, McIntosh M, Atkinson C, et al. Validation of a commercially available indirect assay for SARS-CoV-2 neutralising antibodies using a pseudotyped virus assay. J Infect 2021;82(5):170–7.

23. Santano R, Barrios D, Crispi F, et al. Agreement between commercially available ELISA and in-house Luminex SARS-CoV-2 antibody immunoassays. bioRxiv. Sci Rep 2021. https://doi.org/10.1101/2021.03.09.21252401.

24. Martinaud C, Hejl C, Igert A, et al. Evaluation of the Quotient® MosaiQ™ COVID-19 antibody microarray for the detection of IgG and IgM antibodies to SARS-CoV-2 virus in humans. J Clin Virol 2020;130:104571.

25. Zhu C, Yang G, Li H, et al. Electrochemical sensors and biosensors based on nanomaterials and nanostructures. Anal Chem 2015;87(1):230–49.

26. Chiang SH, Tu M, Cheng J, et al. Development and validation of a highly sensitive and specific electrochemical assay to quantify anti-SARS-CoV-2 IgG antibodies to facilitate pandemic surveillance and monitoring of vaccine response. medRxiv 2020. https://doi.org/10.1101/2020.11.12.20230656.

27. Torrente-Rodríguez RM, Lukas H, Tu J, et al. SARS-CoV-2 RapidPlex: a graphene-based multiplexed telemedicine platform for rapid and low-cost COVID-19 diagnosis and monitoring. Matter 2020;3(6):1981–98.

28. Rashed MZ, Kopechek JA, Priddy MC, et al. Rapid detection of SARS-CoV-2 antibodies using electrochemical impedance-based detector. bioRxiv 2020. https://doi.org/10.1101/2020.08.10.20171652.

29. Ali MA, Hu C, Jahan S, et al. Sensing of COVID-19 antibodies in seconds via aerosol jet nanoprinted reduced-graphene-oxide-coated 3D electrodes. Adv Mater 2021;33(7):e2006647.

30. Yakoh A, Pimpitak U, Rengpipat S, et al. Paper-based electrochemical biosensor for diagnosing COVID-19: detection of SARS-CoV-2 antibodies and antigen. Biosens Bioelectron 2020;176:112912.

31. Burbelo PD, Riedo FX, Morishima C, et al. Sensitivity in detection of antibodies to nucleocapsid and spike proteins of severe acute respiratory syndrome coronavirus 2 in patients with coronavirus disease 2019. J Infect Dis 2020;222(2):206–13.

32. Burbelo PD, Ching KH, Klimavicz CM, et al. Antibody profiling by luciferase immunoprecipitation systems (LIPS). J Vis Exp 2009;(32). https://doi.org/10.3791/1549.

33. Elledge SK, Zhou XX, Byrnes JR, et al. Engineering luminescent biosensors for point-of-care SARS-CoV-2 antibody detection. Nat Biotechnol 2021. https://doi.org/10.1038/s41587-021-00878-8.

34. Huang P-S, Boyken SE, Baker D. The coming of age of de novo protein design. Nature 2016;320–7. https://doi.org/10.1038/nature19946.

35. Quijano-Rubio A, Yeh H-W, Park J, et al. De novo design of modular and tunable protein biosensors. Nature 2021;591(7850):482–7.

36. Dzimianski JV, Lorig-Roach N, O'Rourke SM, et al. Rapid and sensitive detection of SARS-CoV-2 antibodies by biolayer interferometry. Sci Rep 2020;10(1):21738.

37. Sun Y, Fan X. Optical ring resonators for biochemical and chemical sensing. Anal Bioanal Chem 2011;399(1):205–11.

38. Miyara M, Charuel J-L, Mudumba S, et al. Detection in whole blood of autoantibodies for the diagnosis of connective tissue diseases in near patient testing condition. PLoS One 2018;13(8):e0202736.

39. Donato LJ, Theel ES, Baumann NA, et al. Evaluation of the Genalyte Maverick SARS-CoV-2 multi-antigen serology panel. J Clin Virol Plus 2021;100030. https://doi.org/10.1016/j.jcvp.2021.100030.

40. Suhandynata RT, Hoffman MA, Huang D, et al. Commercial serology assays predict neutralization activity against SARS-CoV-2. Clin Chem 2021;67(2):404–14.

41. Luchsinger LL, Ransegnola BP, Jin DK, et al. Serological assays estimate highly variable SARS-CoV-2 neutralizing antibody activity in recovered COVID-19 patients. J Clin Microbiol 2020;58(12). https://doi.org/10.1128/JCM.02005-20.
42. Wang Z, Lorenzi JCC, Muecksch F, et al. Enhanced SARS-CoV-2 neutralization by dimeric IgA. Sci Transl Med 2021;13(577). https://doi.org/10.1126/scitranslmed.abf1555.
43. Hebert CG, Rodrigues KL, DiNardo N, et al. Viral infectivity quantification and neutralization assays using laser force cytology. Methods Mol Biol 2021;2183:575–85.
44. Cantoni D, Mayora-Neto M, Temperton N. The role of pseudotype neutralization assays in understanding SARS CoV-2. Oxf Open Immunol 2021;2(1):iqab005.
45. Vandergaast R, Carey T, Reiter S, et al. Development and validation of IMMUNO-COVTM: a high-throughput clinical assay for detecting antibodies that neutralize SARS-CoV-2. bioRxiv 2020. https://doi.org/10.1101/2020.05.26.117549.
46. Zhang Z, Wang X, Wei X, et al. Multiplex quantitative detection of SARS-CoV-2 specific IgG and IgM antibodies based on DNA-assisted nanopore sensing. Biosens Bioelectron 2021;181:113134.
47. Bhalla N, Pan Y, Yang Z, et al. Opportunities and challenges for biosensors and nanoscale analytical tools for pandemics: COVID-19. ACS Nano 2020;14(7):7783–807.
48. Xu GJ, Kula T, Xu Q, et al. Viral immunology. Comprehensive serological profiling of human populations using a synthetic human virome. Science 2015;348(6239):aaa0698.
49. Soh JH, Chan H-M, Ying JY. Strategies for developing sensitive and specific nanoparticle-based lateral flow assays as point-of-care diagnostic device. Nano Today 2020;30:100831.
50. Dalai SC, Dines JN, Snyder TM, et al. Clinical validation of a novel T-cell receptor sequencing assay for identification of recent or prior SARS-CoV-2 infection. medRxiv 2021. https://doi.org/10.1101/2021.01.06.21249345.
51. Isho B, Abe KT, Zuo M, et al. Persistence of serum and saliva antibody responses to SARS-CoV-2 spike antigens in COVID-19 patients. Sci Immunol 2020;5(52). https://doi.org/10.1126/sciimmunol.abe5511.
52. Pisanic N, Randad PR, Kruczynski K, et al. COVID-19 serology at population scale: SARS-CoV-2-Specific antibody responses in saliva. J Clin Microbiol 2020;59(1). https://doi.org/10.1128/JCM.02204-20.

Suboptimal Humoral Immunity in Severe Acute Respiratory Syndrome Coronavirus 2 Infection and Viral Variant Generation

Shiv Pillai, MBBS, PhD

KEYWORDS

- SARS-CoV-2 • COVID-19 • Humoral immunity • Germinal centers
- T follicular helper cells • Variant generation • Immune pressure

KEY POINTS

- Severe COVID-19 generates neutralizing antibodies but with very little affinity maturation.
- In these patients switched memory B cells are generated extra-follicularly.
- Germinal centers do not properly develop in severe COVID-19.

The existence of novel coronavirus infection in Wuhan China was established in late December 2019.[1,2] The severe acute respiratory disease first documented at that time and now called coronavirus disease (COVID)-19, was in terms of clinical features, virtually indistinguishable from SARS (severe acute respiratory syndrome) observed only in 2002 and 2003.[3] Although there was a delay of many months before the viral etiology of the "original" SARS was finally identified in May 2003, the virus that caused the novel viral disease in Wuhan in 2019 was identified by many laboratories in a matter of days in the last week of 2019. The sequence of this positive orientation, single-stranded enveloped RNA virus bore strong similarities to the SARS coronavirus as well as to the coronavirus that causes a related disease, called Middle East respiratory syndrome or MERS.[4] The virus of the 2002 to 2003 epidemic is now called SARS-CoV (or sometimes SARS-1) and the coronavirus that causes COVID-19 is called SARS-CoV-2.

Although SARS-CoV-2 is clearly more easily transmissible than SARS-CoV, and certainly far more extensive and sophisticated studies have been performed in COVID-19 than were undertaken in SARS, at this point, in terms of the "bigger picture", it does not appear that there are major differences in the overall adaptive

Ragon Institute of MGH, MIT and Harvard, Harvard Medical School, Cambridge, MA 02139, USA
E-mail address: pillai@helix.mgh.harvard.edu

Clin Lab Med 42 (2022) 75–84
https://doi.org/10.1016/j.cll.2021.10.001
0272-2712/22/© 2021 Elsevier Inc. All rights reserved.

labmed.theclinics.com

immune responses seen in COVID-19 than those that were seen in SARS, nor are the changes seen so far in the lung particularly different. However, draining lymph nodes, the sites of adaptive immune response induction, have rarely been systematically interrogated in the context of any human infectious diseases and our studies on COVID-19 focused on the site of severe infection (the lungs) and on secondary lymphoid organs including the draining thoracic lymph nodes and the spleen.

The nature of the T-dependent B cell response in viral infections determines the extent of the durability of the protective antibody response, but T–B interactions in the context of dysregulated inflammation may also contribute to pathologic alterations in B cells and thus to disease progression and disease sequelae. The emergence of B cells with a switched-memory phenotype is not in itself a marker for durability, (the length of time for which there is effective protection from reinfection by circulating antibodies). Memory B cells disappeared during a 6-year follow-up period in patients with SARS.[5] In COVID-19, natural immunity (immunity generated by infection) has been documented to decline and does not effectively generate protection or herd immunity.[6–10] We believe that suboptimal adaptive immunity against SARS-CoV-2 as documented by us in terms of the cells involved in humoral immunity,[11] but which also likely applies to cellular immunity, facilitates viral persistence, and variant generation. In this review, we will first discuss the durability of natural immunity in SARS, MERS, and COVID-19. We will then discuss the biology of germinal centers and the loss of germinal centers in severe COVID-19 and focus on the loss of Bcl-6+ T follicular helper cells in this disease. We will subsequently discuss the loss of germinal centers in other severe infections in animal models and examine what that might suggest in a mechanistic sense. Finally, we will consider the potential pathologic consequences of the extrafollicular B cell response in COVID-19.

NATURAL IMMUNITY IN SEVERE ACUTE RESPIRATORY SYNDROME, MIDDLE EAST RESPIRATORY SYNDROME RARELY GENERATED DURABLE HUMORAL IMMUNITY, AND THE DATA ON CORONAVIRUS DISEASE-19 ARE STILL EMERGING

Slifka, Antia, Ahmed, and colleagues have highlighted the dichotomy between the robust, virtually life-long, humoral immunity seen with natural infections with viruses such as measles, mumps, and rubella or vaccination with live-attenuated viral vaccines (with calculated antibody half-lives ranging roughly from 50 to 100 years) in comparison to the steadily declining humoral immunity seen in most of the infections with SARS and MERS and after immunization with killed parenteral vaccines such as the one used in influenza.[12–15] In one of the deepest follow-up studies in SARS, a disease for which the virus was rapidly eliminated, and no vaccine was administered subsequently, patients were followed for up to 6 years after infection.[5] Virus-specific IgG antibodies steadily waned and had completely disappeared in 21 of 23 patients; specific memory B cells had also become undetectable in all 23 by the end of the study, though about half preserved memory T cells.

In COVID-19, vaccine availability may make conducting a similar study difficult, but all indications are that a trajectory for humoral immunity that is, similar to that observed in SARS is likely. Both antigen-specific switched memory B cells and plasma cells can, therefore, either be relatively short-lived, in the order of 2 to 4 years, after an infection such as SARS, or very long-lived after infection with measles or mumps or after yellow fever vaccination. Just as we recognize that short-lived plasma cells are of extrafollicular origin while long-lived plasma cells emerge from the germinal center, are there 2 different sites at which switched memory B cells are generated after different categories of human viral infections?

Is there an underlying immunologic explanation for why the durability of specific humoral immunity in SARS, MERS, and likely COVID-19 is so different from humoral immunity in infections such as measles, mumps, and rubella? What exactly is the relevance of antigen-specific switched memory B cells in COVID-19? It is also of some interest to ask whether the altered nature of the humoral immune response initiated in the draining lymph nodes in infections such as SARS, MERS, and COVID-19 (and described by us in COVID-19 as discussed in this review) may contribute to a possible increase in disease-related B cells in the end-organ and thus to the pathogenesis of COVID-19.

Most of our understanding of the pathogenesis of severe COVID-19 has been derived from generally nonquantitative studies of the blood, with few systematic studies of adaptive immune cells at the sites of infection and in draining lymph nodes. Although the virus attenuates type I interferon production by infected cells[16,17] and the antiviral state is further compromised in some susceptible individuals by mutations or by preexisting antibodies to type I interferons,[18,19] most of the initial tissue damage in the lungs is likely generated by excessive unregulated inflammation.

THE BIOLOGY OF THE GERMINAL CENTER RESPONSE

One of the most remarkable phenomena in adaptive immunity that has been of great interest to immunologists as well as molecular biologists is the germinal center response. This response is the key to protective responses against most pathogens and is central to the success of vaccination.

Over a century ago, pathologists had recognized the presence of proliferating cells in organized collections in lymph nodes (reviewed in [20]). It had originally been assumed, incorrectly, that these were the sites at which lymphocytes were generated, hence they were called "germinal centers." Little was known then, however, as to what lymphocytes actually did. The function of lymphocytes in adaptive immunity would only be established in 1957 by Gowans.[21] It soon became clear that there were 2 types of lymphocytes. B lymphocytes are generated in the bursa of Fabricius in birds (or the bone marrow in other vertebrates), whereas T lymphocytes are generated in the thymus.[22,23] In the early 1960s, it was eventually recognized that germinal centers were not the sites at which lymphocytes are made. Over the next decade, it became apparent that germinal centers are induced structures that emerge after immunization, but their precise functional role remained mysterious for a while.

Although the increase in the affinity of antibodies after repeated immunization, a phenomenon called affinity maturation had been described well before the function of lymphocytes was appreciated, nothing was known about how this phenomenon occurred until the early 1980s (reviewed in[24,25]). The theoretic possibility that antibody diversity might be caused by a process of somatic mutation had been entertained even in the 1960s by Burnet and others.[26] In the early 1970s, the sequencing of antibodies using Edman degradation started to reveal the theoretic possibilities of somatic mutation in antibody diversification, but whether this phenomenon occurred during lymphocyte development or after an immune response was initiated was not entirely clear. The recombinant DNA revolution in the early 1970s and the subsequent cloning of antibody genes started the process by which the function of the germinal center would begin to be understood in the early 1980s. The crucial molecular descriptions of the process of somatic hypermutation by the early 1980s also depended on the ability to generate single clonal B cells and monoclonal antibodies, a technology originally developed by Kohler and Milstein to better understand somatic hypermutation.

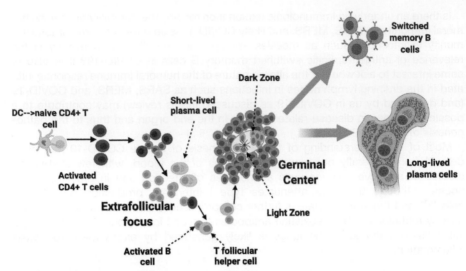

Fig. 1. A schematic overview of germinal center formation and the germinal center response.

The germinal center response is essential for the production of high-affinity antibodies and long-lived plasma cells. It may also contribute to the generation of memory B cells although the requirement for the germinal center for memory B cell generation is not absolute.[27] A current overview of germinal center biology is provided in **Fig. 1.** It summarizes detailed knowledge acquired over many decades about this Darwinian process. During an immune response to a protein antigen, helper T cells that recognize a linear peptide determinant within this protein antigen (and that is presented on MHC class II molecules), collaborate with B cells that see a conformational determinant on the same protein antigen. The initial interaction of these cognate helper T cells and B cells occurs at the interface between the T and B cell zones and leads to T cells activating B cells and inducing an extrafollicular B cell response. This extrafollicular response leads to B cell activation and proliferation, isotype switching to most human isotypes other than IgE, some memory B cell generation, and some differentiation of activated B cells into short-lived plasma cells (reviewed in 24, 25).

Naïve CD4+ T cells are initially activated by specific peptide antigens presented on dendritic cells in the T cell zone, and these cells then migrate toward the B cell zone to activate specific B cells that have migrated to the T–B interface.[28,29] These activated helper T cells that drive the initial extrafollicular activation of B cells are sometimes referred to as pregerminal center T follicular helper cells or pre-GC T_{FH} cells. These cells are not in the follicle, so they are only precursors of "true" T_{FH} cells.[28,29] At the time that the extrafollicular response is generated (or soon after), activated B cells that now express ICOS-L activate some of these previously activated CD4+ helper T cells and induce their polarization into Bcl-6-expressing T follicular helper cells – cells that are sometimes called GC-T_{FH} cells.[11] These cells express high levels of CXCR5 and enter the follicle, likely each with an interacting activated B cell and then set up the germinal center. In the germinal center, B cells proliferate rapidly and undergo somatic hypermutation in a dense region known as the dark zone. After some rounds of proliferation and genetic diversification of the antibody heavy and light chain genes mainly in the regions encoding the V domains, dark zone B cells migrate to the light zone whereby high-affinity B cells recognize antigen held up on follicular dendritic cells. If they successfully capture the protein antigen and present it, they are selected in the light zone by T follicular helper cells. Selected cells return to the dark zone and there are repeated rounds of somatic hypermutation and selection. Unselected B cells die by apoptosis in the light zone. Early in the germinal center reaction memory B cells emerge, though they may also be generated extrafollicularly. After many rounds of selection, B cells are immortalized as plasmablasts that migrate to the bone marrow and differentiate into long-lived plasma cells.

THE LOSS OF GERMINAL CENTERS IN SEVERE CORONAVIRUS DISEASE -19

We have demonstrated the loss of germinal centers in thoracic lymph nodes in severe COVID-19, as shown in **Fig. 2**.[11] A pathologic description consistent with our data has also been reported,.[30] Thoracic lymph nodes, such as Peyer's patches and mesenteric lymph nodes, constitutively contain germinal centers; age-matched elderly individuals who died of non–COVID-19 causes in the same time window (and were autopsied in a similar accelerated manner to those who succumbed to COVID-19) had robust germinal centers presumably induced by protein antigens from microbes or allergens constitutively present in the respiratory tract.[11] The presence of germinal centers in human thoracic lymph nodes is the norm. The loss of germinal centers in COVID-19 and in SARS[11,30,31] is reminiscent of the loss of germinal centers in animal models of severe viral infection[32] and is likely a general phenomenon when the lymph node milieu is altered by high levels of locally expressed cytokines in the context of a severe infection. However, in patients who survive, it is to be expected that with recovery, the lymph node cytokine milieu that prevents T follicular helper cell maturation and germinal center formation will dissipate. The restoration of affinity maturation in some convalescent individuals who have recovered from severe COVID-19 favors such a view.[33]

Quantitation of B cells in the thoracic lymph nodes and the nodes and the spleen showed a dramatic decrease in the absolute numbers as well as percentages of Bcl-6+ CD19+ B cells – basically a loss of germinal center B cells. There was, however, preservation of AID + CD19+ B cells clearly indicating that there was T–B collaboration was preserved both in the follicle and outside the follicle though germinal centers failed to form.[11]

Our previous studies also showed that SARS-CoV-2-specific switched memory B cells were identifiable in the blood of patients with severe COVID-19.[11] These data raised the possibility that the limited durability of humoral responses to some viral infections such as SARS and MERS on the one hand and the extremely long-lived

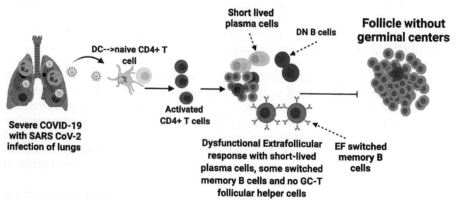

Fig. 2. An overview summary of the failure to generate germinal centers in severe COVID-19.

humoral immunity seen in infections such as measles, mumps, and rubella may have an underlying biological basis, related to the type of memory B cell populations generated in these contexts. In SARS, MERS, and COVID-19, the paucity or absence of proper germinal centers in lymph nodes could result in class-switched memory B cells that develop primarily outside germinal centers, a phenomenon well-established in rodents,[27] but not widely appreciated or studied. It is likely that the durability of memory B cells and plasma cells generated outside the germinal center at extrafollicular sites does not match the durability of their counterparts generated in germinal centers, though this has not been formally studied. Although germinal centers likely recover in a subset of survivors of severe infections as suggested from the studies of Wilson and colleagues,[33] and SARS-CoV-2 infection may persist in the gut in many for at least a few months,[34] long-lived plasma cell generation is likely somewhat compromised in COVID-19, as it likely was in SARS.[5] In diseases such as mumps, rubella, and measles both class-switched memory B cells and long-lived plasma cells are likely generated in germinal centers thus generating much greater durability, typically extending for decades.[13]

LOSS OF BCL-6 EXPRESSING FOLLICULAR HELPER CELLS IN SEVERE CORONAVIRUS DISEASE-19

We showed that in patients with severe COVID-19 lymph node architecture was well preserved, there were well-defined follicles and T cell zones and that most CD4+ T cell subsets and regulatory T cells were well preserved.[11] There was, however, a striking loss of T follicular helper cells, especially Bcl-6+ T follicular helper cells. This loss of Bcl-6+ T follicular helper cells would suffice to explain the loss of germinal center B cells.[11]

We showed that there were high levels of TNF-α expression in the thoracic lymph nodes in severe COVID-19[11] and we postulated that, as had been more mechanistically examined in murine models of severe intracellular infections discussed briefly in the next section, the high levels seen of TNF-α in lymph nodes might account for the loss of germinal centers in severe COVID-19.

THE LOSS OF GERMINAL CENTERS IN ANIMAL MODELS OF SEVERE INTRACELLULAR INFECTIONS

There are a few murine models of intracellular infections in which germinal centers are lost, and in some, a block in T_{FH} cell differentiation has also been observed.[35–37] In a murine malaria model, the loss of T_{FH} cells and germinal centers was observed and this was reversed by the blockade of TNF-α or IFN-γ. Genetic deletion of T-bet also prevented the loss of germinal centers. The T_{FH} cell precursors did not express high levels of PD-1 and CXCR5 but expressed genes such as T-bet and CXCR3, characteristic of T_{H1} cells.[35]

In a study of a murine rickettsial infection caused by *Ehrlichia muris*, the loss of germinal centers was reversed by TNF-α blockade as well as by the use of mice that have an engineered deletion of TNF-α.[36] In another study involving *Salmonella* infection, IL-12 was shown to be responsible for the block in T_{FH} cell differentiation and the loss of germinal centers that was seen.[37] Given the known functional and sequential links between IL-12, T_{H1} cells and the downstream production of TNF-α, we suspect that signaling through TNFRII on CD4+ T cells might cause a block in T_{FH} cell differentiation in these models and in severe viral infections.

There is a slightly artificial murine viral infection model in which germinal centers are lost.[32] When regular inbred mice are first immunized with a specific LCMV peptide that activates CD4+ T cells and then later infected with LCMV clone 13, they develop a severe viral infection that results in lymphopenia, the loss of germinal centers in lymph nodes, and an eventually lethal severe viral infection that involves the lungs and other organs. This disease resembles severe COVID-19 in many ways. Very high levels of IL-12 were observed in these mice. Overall a number of severe intracellular infections result in the loss of germinal centers, and this may involve in some poorly defined way, the sequential induction of high levels of IL-12, IFN-γ, and TNF-α.[11,32,35–37]

THE EXTRAFOLLICULAR B CELL RESPONSE IN CORONAVIRUS DISEASE-19 AND ITS POTENTIAL CONTRIBUTION TO PATHOLOGY

Some activated B cell subsets seem to be key drivers of inflammatory and fibrotic diseases, many of which respond therapeutically to B cell depletion. Our previous studies revealed the presence of subsets of antigen-specific disease-related IgD⁻CD27⁻ double negative (DN) B cells that accumulate in the blood of patients with COVID-19 including those with severe disease[11] and similar overall B cell populations have been observed by others.[38] We have demonstrated that DN B cells in COVID-19 include SARS-CoV-2 specific cells, but there is no definitive evidence as yet that these cells actually produce the large number of autoantibodies now described in patients with COVID-19.[39,40] The presence of these cells B cell in the blood correlates with immune dysregulation and a break in B and T cell tolerance in COVID-19. It has, however, never been established whether DN B cells actually accumulate in the lesions of inflammatory or fibrotic diseases, even in diseases that respond to B cell depletion or if they interact with CD4+ T cells in end-organs. Whether or not specific DN B cell subsets may be more relevant in a tissue context on inflammatory and fibrotic diseases has also not been investigated.

Although the contribution, if any, of B cells to the progression or sequelae of COVID-19 is unclear, the global lack of B cells, however, seems to correlate with less severe COVID-19, and this infection has been reported to be less likely to be lethal in patients with X-linked agammaglobulinemia.[41–43] This could be due to the paucity of B cells in these patients rather or possibly defective BTK signaling in myeloid and lymphoid cells. BTK inhibition seems to reduce hospitalization rates and disease progression in patients with COVID-19[44] though the results of randomized clinical trials are awaited, anti–CD20-mediated B cell depletion has been seen to be clinically useful in ameliorating severe progressive interstitial lung disease[45,46] and also in reversing progression in severe combined immunodeficiency with associated granulomatous-lymphocytic interstitial lung disease.[47] Although there is no consensus view about B cell depletion in COVID-19 (in patients receiving anti-CD20 for other diagnoses), it has frequently been suggested to be beneficial. As no clear-cut negative outcomes have been observed with anti-CD20, trials using this therapeutic in various clinical contexts were allowed to resume in Europe in early 2021.

SUMMARY

Mild COVID-19 generates very poor antibody responses likely because the virus is contained by type I interferons generated by plasmacytoid dendritic cells, is rapidly cleared, and antigen does not accumulate in draining lymph nodes. Affinity maturation is rare with moderate and severe COVID-19, because viral infection results in an altered draining lymph node milieu that impairs GC-T$_{FH}$ cell generation and germinal center formation. In addition, measurable T cell responses have only been observed late in convalescence and the virus persists. In the absence of affinity maturation, immune pressure is undoubtedly suboptimal and most likely is a driver of variant generation.

CLINICS CARE POINTS

- Natural immunity is generated in severe COVID-19 but there is a defect in neutralization breadth.
- Natural immunity may best be supplemented by vaccination as recent studies now suggest.

ACKNOWLEDGMENTS

This work was supported by NIH U19 AI110495 and the Massachusetts Consortium for Pathogen Readiness.

REFERENCES

1. Zhou P, Yang XL, Wang XG, et al. A pneumonia outbreak associated with a new coronavirus of probable bat origin. Nature 2020;579:270–3.
2. Zhu N, Zhang D, Wang W, et al. A novel coronavirus from patients with pneumonia in China, 2019. N Engl J Med 2020;382:727–33.
3. Perlman S, Dandekar AA. Immunopathogenesis of coronavirus infections: implications for SARS. Nat Rev Immunol 2005;5:917–27.
4. Zumla A, Hui DS, Perlman S. Middle east respiratory syndrome. Lancet 2015;386: 995–1007.
5. Tang F, Quan Y, Xin ZT, et al. Lack of peripheral memory B cell responses in recovered patients with severe acute respiratory syndrome: a six-year follow-up study. J Immunol 2011;186:7264–8.
6. Brouwer PJM, Caniels TG, van der Straten K, et al. Potent neutralizing antibodies from COVID-19 patients define multiple targets of vulnerability. Science 2020; 369(6504):643–50.
7. Long QX, Liu BZ, Deng HJ, et al. Antibody responses to SARS-CoV-2 in patients with COVID-19. Nat Med 2020;26:845–8.
8. Robbiani DF, Gaebler C, Muecksch F, et al. Convergent antibody responses to SARS-CoV-2 in convalescent individuals. Nature 2020;584(7821):437–42.
9. Buss LF, Prete CA Jr, Abrahim CMM, et al. Three-quarters attack rate of SARS-CoV-2 in the Brazilian Amazon during a largely unmitigated epidemic. Science 2021;371:288–92.
10. Sridhar D, Gurdasani D. Herd immunity by infection is not an option. Science 2021;371:230–1.
11. Kaneko N, Kuo HH, Boucau J, et al. Loss of Bcl-6-expressing T follicular helper cells and germinal centers in COVID-19. Cell 2020;183:143–157 e113.
12. Ahmed R, Gray D. Immunological memory and protective immunity: understanding their relation. Science 1996;272:54–60.
13. Amanna IJ, Carlson NE, Slifka MK. Duration of humoral immunity to common viral and vaccine antigens. N Engl J Med 2007;357:1903–15.
14. Antia A, Ahmed H, Handel A, et al. Heterogeneity and longevity of antibody memory to viruses and vaccines. Plos Biol 2018;16:e2006601.
15. Davis CW, Jackson KJL, McCausland MM, et al. Influenza vaccine-induced human bone marrow plasma cells decline within a year after vaccination. Science 2020;370:237–41.

16. Blanco-Melo D, Nilsson-Payant BE, Liu WC, et al. Imbalanced host response to SARS-CoV-2 drives development of COVID-19. Cell 2020;181:1036–1045e1039.

17. Hadjadj J, Yatim N, Barnabei L, et al. Impaired type I interferon activity and inflammatory responses in severe COVID-19 patients. Science 2020;369:718–24.

18. Zhang Q, Bastard P, Liu Z, et al. Inborn errors of type I IFN immunity in patients with life-threatening COVID-19. Science 2020a;370(6515):eabd4570.

19. Bastard P, Rosen LB, Zhang Q, et al. Autoantibodies against type I IFNs in patients with life-threatening COVID-19. Science 2020;370(6515):eabd4585.

20. Nieuwenhuis P, Opstelten D. Functional anatomy of germinal centers. Am J Anat 1984;170:421–35.

21. McGregor DD, Gowans JL. The antibody response of rats depleted of lymphocytes by chronic drainage from the thoracic Duct. J Exp Med 1963;117:303–20.

22. Miller JF. Analysis of the thymus influence in leukaemogenesis. Nature 1961;191: 248–9.

23. Glick G, Chang TS, Jaap RG. The bursa of Fabricius and antibody production. Poult Sci 1956;35:224–34.

24. Teng G, Papavasiliou FN. Immunoglobulin somatic hypermutation. Annu Rev Genet 2007;41:107–20.

25. Victora GD, Nussenzweig MC. Germinal centers. Annu Rev Immunol 2012;30: 429–57.

26. Burnet FM. A Darwinian Approach to immunity. Nature 1964;203:451–4.

27. Toyama H, Okada S, Hatano M, et al. Memory B cells without somatic hypermutation are generated from Bcl6-deficient B cells. Immunity 2002;17:329–39.

28. Crotty S. T follicular helper cell differentiation, function, and roles in disease. Immunity 2014;41:529–42.

29. Vinuesa CG, Linterman MA, Yu D, et al. Follicular helper T cells. Annu Rev Immunol 2016;34:335–68.

30. Duan YQ, Xia MH, Ren L, et al. Deficiency of Tfh cells and germinal center in deceased COVID-19 patients. Curr Med Sci 2020;40:618–24.

31. Gu J, Gong E, Zhang B, et al. Multiple organ infection and the pathogenesis of SARS. J Exp Med 2005;202:415–24.

32. Penaloza-MacMaster P, Barber DL, Wherry EJ, et al. Vaccine-elicited CD4 T cells induce immunopathology after chronic LCMV infection. Science 2015;347: 278–82.

33. Dugan HL, Stamper CT, Li L, et al. Profiling B cell immunodominance after SARS-CoV-2 infection reveals antibody evolution to non-neutralizing viral targets. Immunity 2021;54(6):1290–303.e7.

34. Gaebler C, Wang Z, Lorenzi JCC, et al. Evolution of antibody immunity to SARS-CoV-2. Nature 2021;591(7851):639–44.

35. Ryg-Cornejo V, Ioannidis LJ, Ly A, et al. Severe malaria infections impair germinal center responses by inhibiting T follicular helper cell differentiation. Cell Rep 2016;14:68–81.

36. Popescu M, Cabrera-Martinez B, Winslow GM. TNF-alpha contributes to lymphoid tissue disorganization and germinal center B cell suppression during intracellular bacterial infection. J Immunol 2019;203:2415–24.

37. Elsner RA, Shlomchik MJ. IL-12 blocks Tfh cell differentiation during Salmonella infection, thereby contributing to germinal center suppression. Cell Rep 2019; 29:2796–809.e5.

38. Woodruff MC, Ramonell RP, Nguyen DC, et al. Extrafollicular B cell responses correlate with neutralizing antibodies and morbidity in COVID-19. Nat Immunol 2020;21:1506–16.

39. Woodruff MC, Ramonell RP, Lee FE, et al. Broadly-targeted autoreactivity is common in severe SARS-CoV-2 Infection. medRxiv 2020.

40. Wang EY, Mao T, Klein J, et al. Diverse functional autoantibodies in patients with COVID-19. medRxiv 2021;Nature 595:283–8.

41. Quinti I, Lougaris V, Milito C, et al. A possible role for B cells in COVID-19? Lesson from patients with agammaglobulinemia. J Allergy Clin Immunol 2020;146: 211–213 e214.

42. Soresina A, Moratto D, Chiarini M, et al. Two X-linked agammaglobulinemia patients develop pneumonia as COVID-19 manifestation but recover. Pediatr Allergy Immunol 2020;31:565–9.

43. Jin H, Reed JC, Liu STH, et al. Three patients with X-linked agammaglobulinemia hospitalized for COVID-19 improved with convalescent plasma. J Allergy Clin Immunol Pract 2020;8:3594–3596 e3593.

44. Stack M, Sacco K, Castagnoli R, et al. BTK inhibitors for severe acute respiratory syndrome coronavirus 2 (SARS-CoV-2): a systematic review. Clin Immunol 2021; 230(108816). https://doi.org/10.1016/j.clim.2021.108816.

45. Keir GJ, Maher TM, Hansell DM, et al. Severe interstitial lung disease in connective tissue disease: rituximab as rescue therapy. Eur Respir J 2012;40:641–8.

46. Fui A, Bergantini L, Selvi E, et al. Rituximab therapy in interstitial lung disease associated with rheumatoid arthritis. Intern Med J 2020;50:330–6.

47. Ng J, Wright K, Alvarez M, et al. Rituximab monotherapy for common variable immune deficiency-associated granulomatous-lymphocytic interstitial lung disease. Chest 2019;155:e117–21.

Antibody Dynamics and Durability in Coronavirus Disease-19

Adam Zuiani, PhD[a,b,c], Duane R. Wesemann, MD, PhD[a,b,d],*

KEYWORDS

- COVID-19 • Antibodies • IgG • IgA • IgM • Durability • Germinal center
- Plasma cells

KEY POINTS

- IgM, IgG, and IgA raised to SARS-CoV-2 appear concurrently in most COVID-19 cases by 10 days after symptom onset.
- Antibody titers are highest in subjects with severe COVID-19 and antibody therapeutics are most effective when administered early.
- Although IgM and IgA decline to near baseline levels over 3 months, total IgG raised during acute COVID-19 peaks 1 month following symptom onset then declines to a relatively stable plateau after recovery for at least 6 months.
- Neutralizing antibody responses are frequently lower titer and may reach baseline faster than total antibody responses.

INTRODUCTION

COVID-19 has emerged as the greatest global health threat in generations. An unprecedented mobilization of researchers has generated a wealth of data on humoral responses to SARS-CoV-2 within a year of the pandemic's beginning. The rapidly developed understanding of acute-phase antibody induction and medium-term antibody durability in COVID-19 is important at an individual level to inform patient care and a population level to help predict transmission dynamics. In this brief review,

Funded by: NIH grant number(s): AI139538; AI165072. Funding also provided by the Massachusetts Consortium on Pathogen Readiness (MassCPR) and the China Evergrande Group.
[a] Department of Medicine, Division of Allergy and Clinical Immunology, Brigham and Women's Hospital, Harvard Medical School, Boston, MA 02115, USA; [b] Department of Medicine, Division of Genetics, Brigham and Women's Hospital, Harvard Medical School, Boston, MA 02115, USA; [c] BioNTech, Cambridge, MA 02139, USA; [d] Ragon Institute of MGH, MIT, and Harvard, Cambridge, MA 02139, USA
* Corresponding author. Department of Medicine, Division of Allergy and Clinical Immunology, Brigham and Women's Hospital, Harvard Medical School, Boston, MA 02115; Ragon Institute of MGH, MIT, and Harvard, Cambridge, MA 02139.
E-mail address: dwesemann@bwh.harvard.edu

Clin Lab Med 42 (2022) 85–96
https://doi.org/10.1016/j.cll.2021.10.004
0272-2712/22/© 2021 Elsevier Inc. All rights reserved.

we will describe the development and maintenance of antibody responses to immunization and infections generally and the specific antibody dynamics observed for COVID-19. These crucial features of the humoral response have implications for the use of antibody therapeutics against the virus and can inform the likelihood of reinfection of individuals by the virus.

OVERVIEW OF B CELL ACTIVATION AND ANTIBODY RESPONSES

Although there is considerable variation between different infectious diseases and vaccinations, the development of pathogen-specific antibodies follows a similar course in most cases. During a primary exposure, the antibody response is generated through the activation of naïve B cells that have completed development but have not previously been activated. B cell development in the bone marrow produces millions of naïve B cell clones, each bearing a unique antibody generated through a process called V(D)J recombination[1]. Antibodies can be expressed both as secreted molecules and as a membrane form on the surface of B cells called the B cell receptor (BCR). Naïve B cells express antibodies in the form of IgM and circulate through blood to the follicles of secondary lymphoid tissues including lymph nodes, the spleen, and mucosal-associated lymphoid tissues like Peyer's patches. Circulation is continuous until the B cell encounters and binds a foreign antigen recognized by its BCR. After BCR binding, the antigen is internalized, digested, and processed for peptide presentation to CD4 T cells on major histocompatibility II (MHCII) surface proteins. CD4 T cells that recognize the peptide component of the foreign antigen displayed on MHCII will supply "help" in the form of activating cytokines and membrane-expressed ligands for costimulatory receptors on the B cell. Once the B cell receives BCR signal and T cell help, it can follow one of the 2 cardinal paths of differentiation into a dedicated antibody-secreting cell. The first is to migrate out of the follicles and immediately begin producing antibodies by differentiating into plasmablasts and short-lived plasma cells (SLPCs). Plasmablasts and SLPCs relatively rapidly undergo apoptosis and produce a transient "extrafollicular" antibody response. The second is to enter a germinal center, a microanatomical site in the follicle in which an antibody refinement process called affinity maturation occurs. Affinity maturation selects B cells bearing the highest affinity antibodies via competition for T cell help for expansion and differentiation into long-lived plasma cells (LLPCs). LLPCs migrate to the bone marrow, whereby they can survive for years or even decades continuously producing high-affinity antibodies.

Different isotypes of antibody emerge during the B cell activation process via class switch recombination (CSR).[2] In brief, CSR is a DNA recombination process that allows the B cell to convert its antibody from its initial expression as IgM to the other antibody isotypes, IgG, IgE, and IgA. The IgM-encoding exons are excised and replaced with exons for another isotype found downstream on the chromosome. IgM production usually precedes other isotypes from the early extrafollicular antibody responses, as it is the form of antibody expressed by naïve B cells. As B cell activation progresses, CSR occurs, and other isotypes begin to appear. Following the resolution of infection and the death of the SLPCs, pathogen-specific IgM in serum will wane but some pathogen-specific IgG will persist, supplied by the LLPCs in the bone marrow. IgG and other isotype levels thus lag IgM by several days but will eventually rise to become the dominant antibody produced in most cases.

A biphasic antibody response emerges from this activation process (**Fig. 1**). For a primary exposure (without preexisting memory), B cell activation takes at least several days to produce measurable antibody following an infectious challenge in all

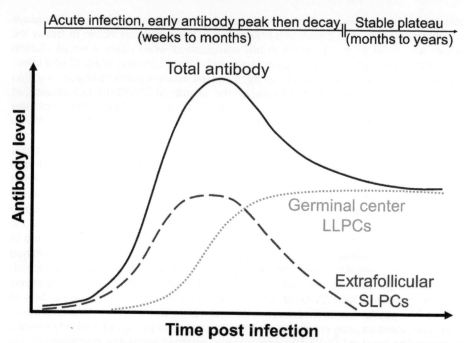

Fig. 1. *Schematic of idealized antibody responses following infection.* A solid purple line represents total antibody levels raised against a pathogen following infection, a dashed red line represents the contribution of extrafollicular SLPCs and plasmablasts and a dotted blue line the contributions of germinal center-originating LLPCs.

circumstances. Peak antibody levels are usually observed several weeks after the initial exposure and are derived from a combination of SLPCs and LLPCs. As the SLPCs undergo apoptosis and the antibodies they produced decay, a stable plateau below the peak is reached representing the contribution of LLPCs. Serum IgG can remain stable for years or even decades with minimal decline assuming robust induction of LLPCs over the course of the infection.

ACUTE PHASE ANTIBODY RESPONSES TO SEVERE ACUTE RESPIRATORY SYNDROME CORONAVIRUS 2

Challenges to Severe Acute Respiratory Syndrome Coronavirus 2 Antibody Research

Studies of antibody responses to SARS-CoV-2 have been published at an unprecedented speed since the beginning of the pandemic; however, several factors can somewhat complicate the synthesis of this collected work into a uniform model of SARS-CoV-2 serology. First, most groups studying SARS-CoV-2 antibodies have used custom assays. Commercially available clinical tests could be used as a universal standard, but they have many limitations including poor quantitation, limited availability at the onset of the pandemic, and high cost to implement. The use of lab-specific assays is particularly an issue with different antigens measured between studies. Usually, a combination of nucleocapsid, spike, and receptor-binding domain of spike is used but rarely are studies exactly identical in the antigen(s) deployed. Also, whether or not the assay used is fully quantitative can affect data interpretation. For instance, many studies use single dilution optical density measures from ELISA assays which are insufficient to generate a true antibody titer; all values above or below the upper and lower limits of detection are compressed when using a single dilution approach. Heterogeneity of disease outcomes observed following SARS-CoV-2 infection influences virus-specific antibody dynamics as different patterns of accumulation and decay may be observed depending on the severity of COVID-19. Individuals that develop symptomatic COVID-19 have a range of experiences from a mild, cold-like disease that resolves in days to lethal pneumonia,[3] Furthermore, 40% to 45% of SARS-CoV-2 individuals are asymptomatically infected, manifesting no symptoms at all following exposure.[4] The patient cohorts used in studies of COVID-19 serology are frequently skewed toward individuals falling into one disease category, and conclusions drawn from these studies may not apply broadly to all COVID-19 cases. Apart from challenges to unifying observations from different studies, a further challenge arises when attempting to relate the speed of SARS-CoV-2 antibody emergence to the time of infection. It would be of great interest to correlate the speed of inducing adaptive immunity to viral clearance. Unfortunately, virtually all studies are limited to timing responses based on time after symptom onset, which can be easily determined by surveys in contrast to determining the specific exposure that resulted in an individual's infection. Because the incubation period before symptom onset is relatively lengthy and varied for COVID-19, ranging from 2 to 14 days with a median of 4 to 5 days,[5,6] time after symptom onset has an uncertain relationship with time after infection. With these caveats in mind, a reasonably consistent picture of antibody kinetics following the onset of COVID-19 symptoms has emerged and will be discussed later in discussion.

Antibody Kinetics During Acute-Phase Coronavirus Disease-19

Early SARS-CoV-2 antibody responses are similar between individuals that ultimately suffer mild disease or moderate to severe disease.[7] A majority of individuals seroconvert between 1- and 2-weeks postsymptom onset.[7-14] Some subjects have been shown to seroconvert before 1 week after symptom onset, but this is uncommon.[8,9,11,12,14,15] By 2 to 3 weeks after symptom onset, greater than 85% of subjects are reported to seroconvert across studies, with many studies reporting close to 100% seroconversion among symptomatic subjects.[8,9,11,13,14,16] With respect to the emergence of different antibody isotypes, humoral immunity in COVID-19 presents interesting deviation from the idealized response detailed above. IgM has not been consistently observed to develop before IgG or IgA in COVID-19; most studies show concurrent development of all 3 isotypes. At approximately 1 month after symptom, onset antibody responses peak in convalescent individuals. The peak antibody response can be robust, but convalescent subjects show a broad range of reported peak titers, with individuals recovering from mild infection (which may still be weeks of symptomatic disease) often showing only modest antibody levels.[17-19] Subjects that fail to swiftly resolve SARS-CoV-2 and develop severe disease continue to accumulate antibody. Disease severity is the most frequently reported correlate of the magnitude of antibody response across many independent studies, with hospitalized subjects consistently reported to have high titer antibody responses.[16-21]

Implications of Severe Acute Respiratory Syndrome Coronavirus 2 Antibody Dynamics for the Use of Antibody Therapeutics

Both convalescent plasma and monoclonal antibody therapeutics were rapidly deployed to treat COVID-19 in the early phases of the pandemic. The absence of anti-SARS-CoV-2 antibodies early after symptom onset and the consistent presence of high titer antibodies in severe COVID-19 suggest that these drugs are most likely to be useful immediately following symptom onset, before endogenous antibody production, and highly unlikely to have a meaningful contribution to disease resolution in individuals with sustained symptoms and/or hospitalization. The available data for both convalescent plasma and monoclonal therapies support this model with the caveat that, in spite of the wide use and reporting on antibody treatment, few rigorous randomized controlled studies (RCTs) have been published. For convalescent plasma, one RCT showed a benefit of treatment within 72 hours after symptom onset to elderly subjects,[22] but 3 other RCTs in which plasma was administered a median of 8 or 9 days after symptom onset showed no difference between control and treatment groups.[23–25] An additional well-conducted retrospective study of convalescent plasma use in COVID-19 supports the administration of high titer plasma to subjects early after symptom onset but found no effect of the treatment later in the disease course.[26] RCT data for monoclonal antibody therapies agree with the results of the convalescent plasma studies. The use of monoclonal therapies for the treatment of hospitalized subjects with severe disease has no demonstrated benefits,[27] whereas the administration of large doses of antibody early following diagnosis has been shown to reduce viral loads and visits to health care facilities.[28–30]

DURABILITY OF SEVERE ACUTE RESPIRATORY SYNDROME CORONAVIRUS 2 ANTIBODY IN CONVALESCENT SUBJECTS
Mixed Longevity of Vaccine- and Infection-Induced Antibodies

The longevity of an antibody response can vary widely. Most infectious challenges or immunizations produce a stable plateau of antibody supplied by LLPCs for many years.[31] However, this durability is not a necessary outcome even following a robust initial antibody response. For example, high titer measles/mumps/rubella (MMR)-vaccine-induced antibodies are estimated to have half-lives in the hundreds or even thousands of years. In contrast, a recent Zika virus vaccine trial showed almost complete loss of initially robust neutralizing antibody responses within 6 months.[32] Understanding whereby COVID-19-induced antibodies fall in this spectrum will influence the interpretation of serology as evidence of past infection and whether herd immunity to SARS-CoV-2 is likely via natural spread alone.

The best viral analogs to help predict COVID-19 antibody durability are related coronaviruses. Seven human disease-causing CoVs have been identified and are divided between 2 genera, the α and β coronaviruses. Two species within each genus are known to cause the common cold, HCoV-229E and HCoV-NL63 among α coronaviruses and HKU.1 and OC43 among β coronaviruses. Insightful data are available for antibody dynamics following HCoV-229E infection from a human challenge study by Callow *and colleagues*.[33] Volunteers were inoculated with HCoV-229E and their antibodies tracked longitudinally, with a secondary viral challenge conducted after 1 year. Antibodies peaked 3-weeks postinfection but then declined to near baseline levels at 1 year. This result suggests that antibody immunity to cold viruses is short-lived, consistent with the reports of rapid reinfection of individuals by these viruses outside of an experimental setting.[34,35] However, a complete loss of antibody to the cold viruses is not likely; in spite of a marked decline. Subjects still had somewhat higher antibody levels 1-year postinfection than in their prechallenge blood draw. Beyond the Callow study, seropositivity for the cold-causing viruses is high across age groups which would be unlikely if antibody was not retained to some extent for greater than 1 year.[36–38]

SARS-CoV and MERS-CoV are β coronaviruses and are the most closely related species to SARS-CoV-2. The available data suggest that antibody durability patterns in both MERS- and SARS-convalescent subjects are similar. Most subjects that have recovered from MERS-CoV-infection seroconvert; however, there is some variability in this regard.[39–42] Individuals that developed pneumonia and recovered display high titer antibody responses, but some individuals with mild or asymptomatic infections fail to produce detectable serum antibody following viral clearance.[39,41] In terms of maintenance of antibody levels, some subjects with mild disease lost detectable serum antibody within a year,[42] but most individuals with symptomatic disease retain detectable antibody for at least 1 year[40–42] and for as long as 3 years.[39] These observations are caveated by a relatively small number of MERS serology studies with low numbers of subjects per study. Seroconversion following SARS-CoV infection occurs between 4 and 14 days after symptom onset for greater than 90% of patients, with subjects developing IgM, IgG, and IgA responses in this window.[43] The durability of SARS-CoV antibodies is well documented,[44–49] with anti-SARS-CoV antibodies peaking 1 to 4 months after symptom onset and decaying to some extent, but not to extinction, by 1 year. Seropositivity is consistently high 2 years following recovery, with studies showing between 88% and 100% IgG positivity in this period.[44–48] However, after 3 years, seropositivity is less reliably observed, ranging from 54% to 100%.[46–48] Antibody levels were low across studies and discrepancies may be explained by differences in assay sensitivity. Additionally, a preprint study has recently reported retention of SARS-CoV antibodies over 12 years, finding that 69% of SARS-convalescent health care worker studies maintained detectable anti-SARS-CoV IgG through this period, albeit at low levels.[49]

Whether antibodies raised during COVID-19 are more similar to responses elicited by common cold-causing HCoVs or SARS-CoV and MERS-CoV is of consequence for projecting the maintenance of immunity and transmission patterns of the virus. However, it should be noted that antibody declines are not always a clear measure of loss of protection. Even if SARS-CoV-2 serum antibody wanes to baseline as observed for HCoV-229E, preexisting antibodies are not the exclusive source of the protection provided by adaptive immunity. Adaptive immune responses also expand pathogen reactive memory B and T cells that can rapidly reactivate upon secondary exposure. In fact, when the Callow HCoV-229E human challenge subjects described above were re-challenged with virus an asymptomatic infection resulted in contrast to their first symptomatic infection, suggesting that memory responses were sufficient to control disease without retention of serum antibody.

Durability of Total Anti-Severe Acute Respiratory Syndrome Coronavirus 2 Antibodies

By the summer of 2020, only a few months into the COVID-19 pandemic, reports of purportedly "rapid" decay of anti-SARS-CoV-2 antibodies were published or posted to the BioRXIV preprint server and widely covered by the popular media. These studies suggested the potential for transient immunity to SARS-CoV-2 following infection, analogous to common cold-causing HCoVs.[33–35] Data are consistent with the biphasic antibody response for anti-SARS-CoV-2 described above in which an initial decay from peak is followed by a lower but stable plateau of IgG.[7,14,18,20,21,50–57] Many studies have tracked the difference between antibody levels at peak, approximately 1 month after symptom onset, and 3 to 4 months later.[18,20,55–57] As expected, IgM rapidly decays in the months following the clearance of SARS-CoV-2, often below the limits of detection, with IgA following a similar trend, suggesting weak induction of IgA-producing LLPCs.[7,9,52,55,56] The IgG response falls from the initial peak to a lower level but very rarely to baseline.[18,20,55–57] Although less data are available for antibody secretion at mucosal sites, one study of antibody levels in saliva suggests that antibodies produced at mucosal surfaces follow a similar pattern to the trends observed in serum.[56] Fewer studies are available looking at later timepoints, but the available data are consistent with stable total anti-SARS-CoV-2 antibody levels after the initial decay, including one rigorous study of adaptive immunity up to 8 months following disease onset.[50,51]

Durability of Severe Acute Respiratory Syndrome Coronavirus 2 Neutralizing Antibody Responses

Antibody levels against viral pathogens can be measured using 2 criteria: the total antibody that binds to viral antigens, most frequently as determined by ELISA, and virus-neutralizing antibody, measured by a neutralization assay. A virus-neutralizing antibody prevents infection by binding to the capsid or envelope proteins on the surface of the virion that facilitates attachment and entry into the host cell. Whereby an ELISA measures the simple binding of an antibody to antigens immobilized on plastic, a neutralization assay measures the capacity of antibodies to block the virus from entering live cells. Neutralization is a more stringent measure than binding alone. Only a subset of the total antibody produced against a virus contributes to neutralization; nonneutralizing antibodies can bind to regions of the viral proteins that do not impact its ability to enter cells. Neutralizing antibody titers correlate strongly with vaccine efficacy against other pathogens. If neutralizing antibodies prove to be critical to protection from SARS-CoV-2 reinfection, tracking retention of neutralizing antibody responses will be key to understanding the persistence of humoral immunity to SARS-CoV-2. Total anti-SARS-CoV-2 antibodies are retained with some decay for at least 6-months postsymptoms onset as described above. However, neutralization may show greater susceptibility to decay as neutralizing antibody levels are lower than total antibody level.[58] Indeed, several studies show a subset of COVID-19 convalescent subjects dropping below the limit of detection for neutralizing antibody as early as 3-months postinfection, while overall seropositivity is almost universally retained.[20,50,51,55,57]

A caveat to these results is that surveys of SARS-CoV-2 neutralizing antibody responses tend to rely on pseudovirus neutralization assays rather than measuring neutralization against authentic SARS-CoV-2 virus. SARS-CoV-2 is designated a biosafety level 3 pathogen, demanding specialized laboratory facilities available only to a few research groups. Pseudoviruses or pseudotyped viruses are chimeric virus particles that bear the surface envelope proteins of one virus, for example, SARS-CoV-2 spike, assembled into a secreted particle using components of another viral species, for example, VSV or HIV. Pseudoviruses do not necessarily incorporate the genetic material needed to replicate and can be used to measure the inhibition of a single round of entry into cells as a surrogate of authentic virus neutralization without posing a risk to researchers. Titers determined using pseudovirus neutralization and live virus neutralization tend to correlate, but are not necessarily identical. An excellent example of discordance between pseudovirus and live virus neutralization can be seen in trial data for the Moderna mRNA-1273 SARS-CoV-2 vaccine for which pseudovirus neutralization seems to underestimate the true neutralizing antibody titer induced by the vaccine as measured using authentic virus assays.[58,59] Additionally, stark discrepancies between pseudovirus- and live virus-measured neutralization for neutralizing monoclonal antibodies targeting the N-terminal domain of the spike protein have been reported, with high potency authentic virus-neutralizing antibodies failing to inhibit pseudovirus entry into cells.[60]

This decay in neutralization occurs in tandem with the emergence of new SARS-CoV-2 variants bearing mutations which reduce the potency of antibody responses raised against the original strain.[61-66] The combination of reduced neutralizing titers and variant strains resistant to antibodies raised against a historically circulating virus may reduce immunity to the virus sufficiently to allow for reinfection, analogous to what has been observed for cold-causing HCoVs.[34,35] The course of the pandemic in the city of Manaus in Brazil may lend credence to this scenario. Manaus had an exceptionally high rate of infection during the first phase of the pandemic in May 2020, with infection rates estimated to be 76% based on a serologic survey.[67] With this infection level, Manaus would be predicted to have achieved herd immunity. However, 8 months following the initial peak, a second COVID-19 wave has leveled a comparable morbidity and mortality burden on the city as a new SARS-CoV-2 variant, P1, swept through Brazil.[68] P1 is known to bear mutations that impact the efficacy of neutralizing antibodies raised against the original Wuhan strain of SARS-CoV-2.[61,63] Further study is necessary to better understand transmission dynamics of SARS-CoV-2 variants through putatively immune populations. Regardless, the prudent course is to deploy the highly efficacious COVID-19 vaccines as widely as possible to ensure robust adaptive immunity is widespread and maintained.

SUMMARY

In summary, antibody responses to SARS-CoV-2 follow a typical biphasic response pattern, reaching a peak approximately 1-month postsymptom onset followed by a period of decay to a stable, months-long plateau. Even following mild COVID-19, SARS-CoV-2 immunity follows a similar pattern to that observed for MERS-CoV or SARS-CoV, reducing the risk of reinfection and disease recurrence upon reexposure to homologous strain virus, as observed for common cold-causing HCoVs. However, genetic drift-driven emergence of new viral variants in tandem with frequently weak neutralizing antibody responses conspires to make reinfection risks with heterologous strains a continued concern. An important goal for future work will be to fully understand heterologous strain reinfection frequencies and to identify the degree to which antibody measurements such as neutralizing levels and SARS-CoV-2 variant cross-reactivity inform predictions and gauge risk levels for disease recurrence.

CLINICS CARE POINTS

- Neutralizing antibody function correlates with total anti-spike IgG levels.
- Neutralizing antibody levels correlates with immune fitness against SARS-CoV-2.
- Assays differ in standardization–requiring caution in interpretation across platforms.
- Protection from SARS-CoV-2 variants likely require greater anti-original-spike antibody levels.

REFERENCES

1. Jung D, Giallourakis C, Mostoslavsky R, et al. Mechanism and control of V(D)J recombination at the immunoglobulin heavy chain locus. Annu Rev Immunol 2006;24(D):541–70.
2. Stavnezer J, Guikema JEJ, Schrader CE. Mechanism and regulation of class switch recombination. Annu Rev Immunol 2008;26:261–92.

3. Wu Z, McGoogan JM. Characteristics of and important lessons from the coronavirus disease 2019 (COVID-19) outbreak in China: summary of a report of 72314 cases from the Chinese center for disease control and prevention. JAMA 2020; 323(13):1239–42.
4. Oran DP, Topol EJ. Prevalence of asymptomatic SARS-CoV-2 infection. Ann Intern Med 2020;173(5):362–7.
5. Lauer SA, Grantz KH, Bi Q, et al. The incubation period of coronavirus disease 2019 (CoVID-19) from publicly reported confirmed cases: Estimation and application. Ann Intern Med 2020;172(9):577–82.
6. Guan W, Ni Z, Hu Y, et al. Clinical Characteristics of Coronavirus Disease 2019 in China. N Engl J Med 2020;382:1708–20. https://doi.org/10.1056/NEJMoa 2002032.
7. Röltgen K, Powell AE, Wirz OF, et al. Defining the features and duration of antibody responses to SARS-CoV-2 infection associated with disease severity and outcome. Sci Immunol 2021;5(54):1–20.
8. Iyer AS, Jones FK, Nodoushani A, et al. Persistence and decay of human antibody responses to the receptor binding domain of SARS-CoV-2 spike protein in COVID-19 patients. Sci Immunol 2020;5(52):1–13.
9. Jiang XL, Wang GL, Zhao XN, et al. Lasting antibody and T cell responses to SARS-CoV-2 in COVID-19 patients three months after infection. Nat Commun 2021;12(1):1–10.
10. Premkumar L, Segovia-Chumbez B, Jadi R, et al. The receptor-binding domain of the viral spike protein is an immunodominant and highly specific target of antibodies in SARS-CoV-2 patients. Sci Immunol 2020;5(48):1–10.
11. Prévost J, Gasser R, Beaudoin-Bussières G, et al. Cross-sectional Evaluation of humoral responses against SARS-CoV-2 spike. Cell Rep Med 2020;1(7):100126.
12. Sterlin D, Mathian A, Miyara M, et al. IgA dominates the early neutralizing antibody response to SARS-CoV-2. medRxiv 2020;2223:eabd2223.
13. Ma H, Zeng W, He H, et al. Serum IgA, IgM, and IgG responses in COVID-19. Cell Mol Immunol 2020;17(7):773–5.
14. Ripperger TJ, Uhrlaub JL, Watanabe M, et al. Orthogonal SARS-CoV-2 serological assays enable surveillance of low-prevalence communities and reveal durable humoral immunity. Immunity 2020;53(5):925–33.e4.
15. Fu Y, Pan Y, Li Z, et al. The utility of specific antibodies against SARS-CoV-2 in laboratory diagnosis. Front Microbiol 2021;11:603058.
16. Long QX, Liu BZ, Deng HJ, et al. Antibody responses to SARS-CoV-2 in patients with COVID-19. Nat Med 2020;26(6):845–8.
17. Robbiani DF, Gaebler C, Muecksch F, et al. Convergent antibody responses to SARS-CoV-2 in convalescent individuals. Nature 2020;584(7821):437–42.
18. Chen Y, Zuiani A, Fischinger S, et al. Quick COVID-19 healers sustain anti-SARS-CoV-2 antibody production. Cell 2020;183(6):1496–507.e16.
19. Bartsch YC, Wang C, Zohar T, et al. Humoral signatures of protective and pathological SARS-CoV-2 infection in children. Nat Med 2021;27(3):454–62.
20. Seow J, Graham C, Merrick B, et al. Longitudinal observation and decline of neutralizing antibody responses in the three months following SARS-CoV-2 infection in humans. Nat Microbiol 2020;5(12):1598–607.
21. Pradenas E, Trinité B, Urrea V, et al. Stable neutralizing antibody levels 6 months after mild and severe COVID-19 episodes. Med 2021;2(3):313–20.e4.
22. Libster R, Pérez Marc G, Wappner D, et al. Early high-titer plasma therapy to prevent severe Covid-19 in older adults. N Engl J Med 2021;384(7):610–8.

23. Simonovich VA, Burgos Pratx LD, Scibona P, et al. A randomized trial of convalescent plasma in covid-19 severe pneumonia. N Engl J Med 2021;384(7): 619–29.

24. Horby PW, Estcourt L, Peto L, et al. Convalescent plasma in patients admitted to hospital with COVID-19 (RECOVERY): a randomised, controlled, open-label, platform trial. medRxiv 2021. 2021.03.09.21252736. Available at: http://medrxiv.org/content/early/2021/03/10/2021.03.09.21252736.abstract.

25. Agarwal A, Mukherjee A, Kumar G, et al. Convalescent plasma in the management of moderate covid-19 in adults in India: open label phase II multicentre randomised controlled trial (PLACID Trial). BMJ 2020;371:1–10.

26. Joyner MJ, Carter RE, Senefeld JW, et al. Convalescent plasma antibody levels and the risk of death from covid-19. N Engl J Med 2021;384(11):1015–27.

27. A neutralizing monoclonal antibody for hospitalized patients with covid-19. N Engl J Med 2021;384(10):905–14.

28. Weinreich DM, Sivapalasingam S, Norton T, et al. REGN-COV2, a neutralizing antibody cocktail, in outpatients with covid-19. N Engl J Med 2021;384(3): 238–51.

29. Chen P, Nirula A, Heller B, et al. SARS-CoV-2 neutralizing antibody LY-CoV555 in outpatients with covid-19. N Engl J Med 2021;384(3):229–37.

30. Gottlieb RL, Nirula A, Chen P, et al. Effect of bamlanivimab as monotherapy or in combination with etesevimab on viral load in patients with mild to moderate COVID-19: a randomized clinical trial. JAMA 2021;325(7):632–44.

31. Amanna IJ, Carlson NE, Slifka MK. Duration of humoral immunity to common viral and vaccine antigens. N Engl J Med 2007;357(19):1903–15.

32. Stephenson KE, Tan CS, Walsh SR, et al. Safety and immunogenicity of a Zika purified inactivated virus vaccine given via standard, accelerated, or shortened schedules: a single-centre, double-blind, sequential-group, randomised, placebo-controlled, phase 1 trial. Lancet Infect Dis 2020;20(9):1061–70.

33. Callow KA, Parry HF, Sergeant M, et al. The time course of the immune response to experimental coronavirus infection of man. Epidemiol Infect 1990;105(2): 435–46. Available at: https://pubmed.ncbi.nlm.nih.gov/2170159.

34. Kiyuka PK, Agoti CN, Munywoki PK, et al. Human coronavirus NL63 molecular epidemiology and evolutionary patterns in rural coastal Kenya. J Infect Dis 2018;217(11):1728–39.

35. Edridge AWD, Kaczorowska J, Hoste ACR, et al. Seasonal coronavirus protective immunity is short-lasting. Nat Med 2020;26(11):1691–3.

36. Gorse GJ, Patel GB, Vitale JN, et al. Prevalence of antibodies to four human coronaviruses is lower in nasal secretions than in serum. Clin Vaccin Immunol 2010; 17(12):1875–80.

37. Shao X, Guo X, Esper F, et al. Seroepidemiology of group I human coronaviruses in children. J Clin Virol 2007;40(3):207–13.

38. Severance EG, Bossis I, Dickerson FB, et al. Development of a nucleocapsid-based human coronavirus immunoassay and estimates of individuals exposed to coronavirus in a U.S. metropolitan population. Clin Vaccin Immunol 2008; 15(12):1805–10.

39. Okba NMA, Raj VS, Widjaja I, et al. Sensitive and specific detection of low-level antibody responses in mild middle east respiratory syndrome coronavirus infections. Emerg Infect Dis J 2019;25(10):1868. Available at: https://wwwnc.cdc.gov/eid/article/25/10/19-0051_article.

40. Payne DC, Iblan I, Rha B, et al. Persistence of antibodies against middle east respiratory syndrome coronavirus. Emerg Infect Dis 2016;22(10):1824–6.

41. Choe PG, Perera RAPM, Park WB, et al. MERS-CoV antibody responses 1 year after symptom onset, South Korea, 2015. Emerg Infect Dis 2017;23(7):1079–84.

42. Alshukairi AN, Khalid I, Ahmed WA, et al. Antibody response and disease severity in healthcare worker MERS survivors. Emerg Infect Dis 2016;22(6):1113–5.

43. Hsueh PR, Huang LM, Chen PJ, et al. Chronological evolution of IgM, IgA, IgG and neutralisation antibodies after infection with SARS-associated coronavirus. Clin Microbiol Infect 2004;10(12):1062–6.

44. Mo H, Zeng G, Ren X, et al. Longitudinal profile of antibodies against SARS-coronavirus in SARS patients and their clinical significance. Respirology 2006; 11(1):49–53.

45. Liu W, Fontanet A, Zhang PH, et al. Two-year prospective study of the humoral immune response of patients with severe acute respiratory syndrome. J Infect Dis 2006;193(6):792–5.

46. Cao W-C, Liu W, Zhang P-H, et al. Disappearance of antibodies to SARS-associated coronavirus after recovery. N Engl J Med 2007;357(11):1162–3.

47. Wu LP, Wang NC, Chang YH, et al. Duration of antibody responses after severe acute respiratory syndrome. Emerg Infect Dis 2007;13(10):1562–4.

48. Liu L, Xie J, Sun J, et al. Longitudinal profiles of immunoglobulin G antibodies against severe acute respiratory syndrome coronavirus components and neutralizing activities in recovered patients. Scand J Infect Dis 2011;43(6–7):515–21.

49. Guo X, Guo Z, Duan C, et al. Long-term persistence of IgG antibodies in SARS-CoV infected healthcare workers. medRxiv 2020.

50. Gaebler C, Wang Z, Lorenzi JCC, et al. Evolution of antibody immunity to SARS-CoV-2. Nature 2021;591. https://doi.org/10.1038/s41586-021-03207-w.

51. Dan JM, Mateus J, Kato Y, et al. Immunological memory to SARS-CoV-2 assessed for up to 8 months after infection. Science 2021;371(6529):eabf4063.

52. Rodda LB, Netland J, Shehata L, et al. Functional SARS-CoV-2-specific immune memory persists after mild COVID-19. Cell 2021;184(1):169–83.e17.

53. Wajnberg A, Amanat F, Firpo A, et al. Robust neutralizing antibodies to SARS-CoV-2 infection persist for months. Science 2020;370(6521):1227–30.

54. Sakharkar M, Rappazzo CG, Wieland-Alter WF, et al. Prolonged evolution of the human B cell response to SARS-CoV-2 infection. Sci Immunol 2021;6(56):1–15.

55. Marot S, Malet I, Leducq V, et al. Rapid decline of neutralizing antibodies against SARS-CoV-2 among infected healthcare workers. Nat Commun 2021;12(1):1–7.

56. Isho B, Abe KT, Zuo M, et al. Persistence of serum and saliva antibody responses to SARS-CoV-2 spike antigens in COVID-19 patients. Sci Immunol 2020; 5(52):1–21.

57. Harrington WE, Trakhimets O, Andrade DV, et al. Rapid decline of neutralizing antibodies is associated with decay of IgM in adults recovered from mild COVID-19 disease. Cell Rep Med 2021;100253. Available at: http://www.ncbi.nlm.nih.gov/pubmed/33842901%0Ahttp://www.pubmedcentral.nih.gov/articlerender.fcgi?artid=PMC8020863.

58. Jackson LA, Anderson EJ, Rouphael NG, et al. An mRNA vaccine against SARS-CoV-2 — preliminary report. N Engl J Med 2020;383(20):1920–31.

59. Doria-Rose N, Suthar MS, Makowski M, et al. Antibody persistence through 6 Months after the second dose of mRNA-1273 vaccine for covid-19. N Engl J Med 2021. https://doi.org/10.1056/NEJMc2103916.

60. Chi X, Yan R, Zhang J, et al. A neutralizing human antibody binds to the N-terminal domain of the Spike protein of SARS-CoV-2. Science 2020;369(6504):650–5.

61. Garcia-Beltran WF, Lam EC, St. Denis K, et al. Multiple SARS-CoV-2 variants escape neutralization by vaccine-induced humoral immunity. Cell 2021;1–12. https://doi.org/10.1016/j.cell.2021.03.013.

62. Chen RE, Zhang X, Case JB, et al. Resistance of SARS-CoV-2 variants to neutralization by monoclonal and serum-derived polyclonal antibodies. Nat Med 2021; 27(4):717–26.

63. Hoffmann M, Arora P, Groß R, et al. SARS-CoV-2 variants B.1.351 and P.1 escape from neutralizing antibodies. Cell 2021;184(9):2384–93.e12.

64. Li Q, Nie J, Wu J, et al. SARS-CoV-2 501Y.V2 variants lack higher infectivity but do have immune escape. Cell 2021;1–10. https://doi.org/10.1016/j.cell.2021.02.042.

65. Planas D, Bruel T, Grzelak L, et al. Sensitivity of infectious SARS-CoV-2 B.1.1.7 and B.1.351 variants to neutralizing antibodies. Nat Med 2021. https://doi.org/10.1038/s41591-021-01318-5.

66. Wang P, Nair MS, Liu L, et al. Antibody resistance of SARS-CoV-2 variants B.1.351 and B.1.1.7. Nature 2021;2021. https://doi.org/10.1038/s41586-021-03398-2.

67. Buss LF, Prete CA, Abrahim CMM, et al. Three-quarters attack rate of SARS-CoV-2 in the Brazilian Amazon during a largely unmitigated epidemic. Science 2021; 371(6526):288–92.

68. Sabino EC, Buss LF, Carvalho MPS, et al. Resurgence of COVID-19 in Manaus, Brazil, despite high seroprevalence. Lancet 2021;397(10273):452–5.

Severe Acute Respiratory Syndrome Coronavirus 2 Antigens as Targets of Antibody Responses

Alana F. Ogata, PhD[a,b,c], Roey Lazarovits, BS[a,b],
Augusta Uwamanzu-Nna, BS[a], Tal Gilboa, PhD[a,b,c],
Chi-An Cheng, PhD[a,b,c], David R. Walt, PhD[a,b,c],*

KEYWORDS

- SARS-CoV-2 • Coronavirus antigens • Antigen-antibody responses
- Humoral immunity

KEY POINTS

- Studies on humoral responses to severe acute respiratory syndrome coronavirus 2 (SARS-CoV-2) antigens have been reported and commonly focus on antibodies targeting spike (S), nucleocapsid (N), and the receptor-binding domain (RBD; anti-S, anti-N, and anti-RBD).
- During acute infection of COVID-19, anti-S and anti-N antibodies have been measured to monitor seroconversion in COVID-19 individuals.
- Anti-RBD immunoglobulin G (IgG), IgM, and IgA antibodies are highly specific to SARS-CoV-2 and show correlation with neutralization assays.
- Unique antibody responses to SARS-CoV-2 antigens show correlation with clinical outcomes and can be used as predictors for disease severity.
- Antibody levels (IgG) lasting several months after infection have been observed, and seropositive individuals (typically determined by anti-SARS-CoV-2 IgG enzyme-linked immunosorbent assays) exhibit protection from reinfection.

BACKGROUND
Severe Acute Respiratory Syndrome Coronavirus 2 Antigens

The novel severe acute respiratory syndrome coronavirus 2 (SARS-CoV-2) was first identified in Wuhan, China in December 2019.[1] SARS-CoV-2 belongs to the Coronaviridae family, which includes Letovirinae and Coronavirinae viruses, which are commonly known as coronaviruses. Coronaviruses are spherical envelope viruses (40–60 nm in

[a] Department of Pathology, Brigham and Women's Hospital, 75 Francis St, Boston, MA 02215, USA; [b] Wyss Institute for Biologically Inspired Engineering, 3 Blackfan Cir, Harvard University, Boston, MA 02115, USA; [c] Harvard Medical School, 25 Shattuck St, Boston, MA 02115, USA
* Corresponding author. 60 Fenwood Road, Boston, MA 02116.
E-mail address: dwalt@bwh.harvard.edu

Clin Lab Med 42 (2022) 97–109
https://doi.org/10.1016/j.cll.2021.10.002
0272-2712/22/© 2021 Elsevier Inc. All rights reserved.

labmed.theclinics.com

responses to SARS-CoV-2 in 63 symptomatic patients from hospitals in China. Upon COVID-19 diagnosis, patients were monitored for IgM and IgG using magnetic chemiluminescence enzyme immunoassays (MCLIA). Recombinant peptides from the SARS-CoV-2 S and N proteins served as targets for antibody detection. Of patients, 98.6% achieved seroconversion, as defined by the first positive test result for IgM or IgG. In a cohort of 63 confirmed COVID-19 participants, 26 initially seronegative individuals were monitored over time and reached seroconversion within 20 days of symptom onset via synchronous seroconversion (simultaneous seroconversion of IgG and IgM) or asynchronous seroconversion (seroconversion of IgM or IgG first, followed by seroconversion of the second immunoglobulin). Guo and colleagues[16] studied symptomatic patients composed of 82 confirmed COVID-19 cases and 58 probable cases (negative quantitative polymerase chain reaction [PCR] result but presented with COVID-19 symptoms) and observed asynchronous seroconversion for anti-N IgG, IgA, and IgM antibodies. IgM and IgA were detected on average 5 days after symptom onset, whereas IgG was detected 14 days after symptom onset. Asynchronous seroconversion is commonly observed for other respiratory viral infections, whereby IgM antibodies are produced first during infection, followed by strong mucosal IgA responses and production of IgG.[18] To assess seroconversion in asymptomatic cases, Long and colleagues obtained 2088 samples from COVID-19 individuals who traveled from Wuhan City or Hubei Province, received a positive reverse transcription (RT)-PCR test, and were quarantined.[19] Thirty-seven individuals were selected as asymptomatic cases, as defined by individuals with a positive RT-PCR test and no clinical symptoms preceding and during hospitalization, for further study, and plasma samples were collected 3 to 4 weeks after the initial positive RT-PCR test and analyzed by MCLIA. In these asymptomatic individuals, 81.1% tested positive for anti-S and anti-N IgG antibodies, and 62.2% tested positive for anti-S and anti-N IgM antibodies. However, anti-S and anti-N IgG levels in asymptomatic individuals were significantly lower than symptomatic individuals. Grzelak and colleagues[17] measured anti-S and anti-N IgG antibodies with 4 serologic assays: an anti-S enzyme linked immunosorbent assay (ELISA), an anti-N ELISA, an S-flow assay, and a luciferase immunoprecipitation system assay in 491 healthy controls, 51 hospitalized COVID-19 patients, and 209 suspected COVID-19 individuals with mild symptoms. The percentage of seropositive samples in hospitalized COVID-19 patients was on average 69% across the 4 serologic assays. Seroconversion in a subset of hospitalized patients was detectable between 5 and 10 days after symptom onset. In comparison, an average of 31% of suspected mild COVID-19 patients tested positive for IgG. The investigators attributed low seropositive rates to low viral loads in mild cases that elicited low antibody responses and analysis of samples collected before an individual seroconverted. Of note, determination of seroconversion is limited by assay sensitivity, which can account for discrepancies in reported seroconversion rates when different serologic methods are used. Nonetheless, these data demonstrate that anti-S and anti-N antibodies can be used to identify current and previous SARS-CoV-2 infections and present evidence that humoral responses are dependent on disease severity.

After observing that SARS-CoV-2 anti-N and anti-S antibody responses differed between symptomatic and asymptomatic individuals, antibodies and their role in clinical outcomes were widely studied. Guthmiller and colleagues[20] studied SARS-CoV-2 anti-S and anti-N antibody responses in 35 acutely infected and 105 convalescent individuals using ELISA. Severe infection was associated with enhanced anti-S and anti-N antibody responses, and high anti-N titers were especially observed in patients who were hospitalized for long durations. Legros and colleagues[21] observed that disease severity, indicated by hospital admission status: outpatient, hospitalized floor, or hospitalized intensive care unit (ICU), strongly correlated with high levels of anti-S1 titers in a cohort of 140 patients. In addition, anti-S IgG antibody measurements and neutralization activity measurements showed that no neutralizing antibodies were present in 3% of hospitalized ICU patients, 34% of hospitalized floor patients, and 70.7% of outpatients. Atyeo and colleagues[22] used bead-based assays to investigate COVID-19 serologic markers in a discovery cohort (N = 22) from Seattle and in a validation cohort (N = 40) from Boston and observed divergent humoral responses between convalescent and deceased individuals. Anti-S IgG1, IgA1, and IgM levels were elevated among convalescent patients, whereas anti-N IgG levels were enhanced in deceased patients (**Fig. 2**A). Deceased patients also showed a less coordinated humoral response (**Fig. 2**B) compared with convalescent individuals who showed coordination between antibodies, natural killer cells, and phagocytic activity. The relationship between antibody responses and COVID-19 severity shows the potential of humoral immunity as a factor in patient care or therapeutic development.

Antibody responses to the receptor-binding domain

As high-resolution data on SARS-CoV-2 epitopes were obtained, RBD showed highly divergent sequences from other human coronaviruses and was identified as a primary target for antibody neutralization in animal models.[23] Premkumar and colleagues[24] developed a sensitive antibody ELISA against the SARS-CoV-2 RBD that had negligible cross-reactivity with antibodies against other human coronavirus RBD. Anti-RBD ELISAs for IgG and IgM were validated in sera from 63 symptomatic COVID-19 patients collected at least 9 days after symptom onset, demonstrating 98% and 81% sensitivity for IgG and IgM, respectively. The investigators then measured anti-RBD IgG, IgM, and IgA antibodies in 48 longitudinal serum samples and showed that most individuals seroconverted for IgG between days 7 and 9 after symptom onset. In addition, anti-RBD titers strongly correlated with SARS-CoV-2 luciferase neutralization assays, whereby 91% of patients showed detectable levels of neutralizing antibodies 21 days after symptom onset. Corroborating studies by Cao and colleagues,[25] Rydyznski Moderbacher and colleagues,[26] and Garcia-Beltran and colleagues[27] showed that neutralizing antibodies are predominantly specific to RBD, and a recent report demonstrated the potential of using commercial anti-RBD assays as a surrogate marker for neutralization.[28] Anti-RBD antibodies also serve as optimal targets in serologic diagnostics, providing high sensitivity and specificity in the detection of immunoglobulins.[6,29,30]

Because of the high correlation between anti-RBD antibodies and SARS-CoV-2 neutralization,[27,31,32] anti-RBD antibodies can provide more sensitive measurements of disease severity compared with anti-S and anti-N antibodies.[27,33,34] Li and colleagues[35] measured anti-S, anti-N, and anti-RBD IgG and IgM antibodies using MCLIA in 1850 patients with severe and mild COVID-19 progression. Recovered COVID-19 patients showed high anti-RBD and anti-S IgG levels. Lower anti-S, anti-RBD, and anti-N levels were associated with longer duration of infection as determined by persistent viral shedding. Röltgen and colleagues[31] similarly observed elevated anti-RBD-to-anti-N ratios in mild individuals compared with severely ill patients. In contrast, Ravichandran and colleagues[33] detected high IgA antibody titers in all patients with severe COVID-19. Anti-RBD IgA was especially high in patients who succumbed to the disease, compared with patients who recovered. Discrepancies in reported antigen-antibody correlations with clinical outcomes may be due to differences in cohort characteristics, whereby age, ethnicity, and geography can influence humoral immunity in a cohort. In addition, time of sampling is critical to determine the

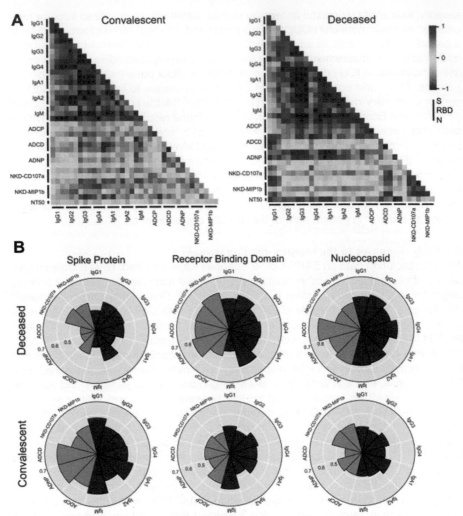

Fig. 2. Deceased individuals showed less coordinated and N-directed antibody responses. (A) The correlation heatmap shows pairwise Spearman correlation matrices of antigen-specific antibody titers and effector functions for convalescent (*left*) and deceased (*right*) patients. For each feature analyzed, the bar covers the S, RBD, and N antigens, shown in the legend on the right. Statistical significance is indicated by gray asterisks with Holm-Bonferroni correction for multiple hypothesis testing (P<.001). Negative correlations are indicated in blue, and positive correlations are denoted in red. (B) The Nightingale Rose plots show the mean percentile of antibody features within the deceased (*top*) and convalescent (*bottom*) groups. Plots represent the S-, RBD-, and N-specific responses across deceased (*top*) and convalescent (*bottom*) individuals. Each wedge represents an SARS-CoV-2 antibody feature. The size of the wedge depicts the magnitude of the value. The colors represent the type of feature: orange, antibody functions; purple, antibody isotypes and subclasses. (*From* Lumley, S. F. *et al.* Antibody Status and Incidence of SARS-CoV-2 Infection in Health Care Workers. *N. Engl. J. Med.* 384, 533–540 (2021); with permission)

sensitivity of antibody tests, as recent analysis of patients who presented early or delayed seroconversion showed no correlation between antibody levels and disease prognosis.[36] Therefore, if individuals exhibit a wide range of seroconversion kinetics, SARS-CoV-2 antibody measurements in samples collected at a single time point after symptom onset may be challenging to interpret.

High-resolution kinetics of antigen-antibody responses

Sensitive antibody detection at early stages of infection is critical for assessing sero-conversion and understanding kinetics of the humoral response. Norman and colleagues[37] demonstrated high-resolution detection of 12 SARS-CoV-2 antibody-antigen interactions during early infection (between zero and 14 days after a positive RT-PCR test) using ultrasensitive single molecule array (Simoa) assays. Simoa enables extremely low limits of detection such that plasma samples were diluted 4000-fold for serologic measurements, which reduced nonspecific binding compared with typical 200-fold dilutions used in ELISA formats. The investigators measured anti-S, anti-S1, anti-RBD, and anti-N IgG, IgM, and IgA responses in longitudinal plasma samples from 4 COVID-19 patients, which showed distinct immune responses. Some patients showed elevated antibody levels 5 days after a positive RT-PCR test[37] (**Fig. 3**A and 3B), whereas others did not mount antibody responses to any antigens after 2 weeks (**Fig. 3**C and 3D). Observation of diverse antibody kinetics among COVID-19 patients was later corroborated by Ogata and colleagues[38] in longitudinal studies of 39 COVID-19 patients. Ogata and colleagues showed that SARS-CoV-2 S, S1, and N antigens were detectable in the blood of severe COVID-19 patients. Antigens were detectable within zero to 10 days after a positive RT-PCR test. Antigen-positive patients showed seroconversion on an average of 7 days after the first positive RT-PCR test, and production of anti-S, anti-S1, and anti-N IgGs, IgAs, and IgMs correlated with S1 and N viral antigen clearance. Although an abundance of antibodies correlates with disease severity, timing of antibody production has also been demonstrated as an indicator of clinical outcome. Lucas and colleagues[39] analyzed 209 patient serum samples and demonstrated that patients who produced anti-RBD antibodies within 14 days of symptom onset correlated with lower mortality compared with those who seroconverted after 14 days. Mechanisms that cause delayed seroconversion remain to be studied. Nonetheless, these data highlight the potential for antibody kinetics and timing of seroconversion as a guide for patient care.

Antigen-Antibody Responses in COVID-19 Pediatric Patients

Clinical manifestations of SARS-CoV-2 differ in adult and pediatric patients. Adults present severe respiratory symptoms, whereas children are often asymptomatic during acute infection. Although many adults and children with COVID-19 become sero-positive, children can develop a novel disease known as multisystem inflammatory syndrome in children (MIS-C) weeks after acute COVID-19 infection and present life-threatening symptoms, such as fever, myocardial disfunction, and cardiogenic shock. Such discrimination between clinical manifestations has been correlated with distinct antibody responses in adult versus pediatric patients. A recent study by Bartsch and colleagues[34] compared SARS-CoV-2 antibody titers in 25 mild COVID-19 pediatric patients, 17 pediatric patients who developed MIS-C, 34 mild COVID-19 adults patients, and 26 severe COVID-19 adult patients. Anti-S, anti-RBD, and anti-N IgM, IgG, and IgA levels were highest in adults with severe COVID-19 and significantly lower in mild COVID-19 adults and both pediatric cohorts. Interestingly, pediatric patients seroconverted earlier than adults with mild illness. However, less pronounced antibody levels suggest that children might not make an effective

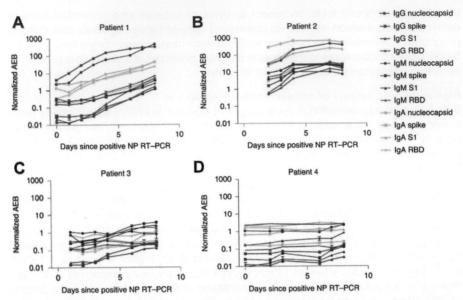

Fig. 3. Profiling the seroconversion time course in COVID-19 patients. (*A–D*) Normalized average number of enzymes per bead (AEB) over the 10 days since a positive nasopharyngeal RT-PCR for patients 1 (*A*), 2 (*B*), 3 (*C*), and 4 (*D*). Patient 1 was a 67-year-old man who recovered 10 days after diagnosis with COVID-19. Patient 2 was a 50-year-old man with multiple comorbidities who died of ARDS 20 days after diagnosis with COVID-19. He received remdesivir from days 1 to 5. Patient 3 was a 50-year-old man with pancytopenia and B-cell acute lymphoblastic leukemia. He died of ARDS 8 days after diagnosis with COVID-19. Patient 4 was an 89-year-old man who died of hypoxemic respiratory failure 8 days after diagnosis with COVID-19. He received hydroxychloroquine from days 1 to 5. The circle, square, triangle, and star represent the mean of 2 replicate measurements, whereas the error bars represent the standard deviation. (*From* Norman, M. *et al.* Ultrasensitive high-resolution profiling of early seroconversion in patients with COVID-19. *Nat. Biomed. Eng.* 4, 1180–1187 (2020); *with permission*.)

humoral response compared with adults. To assess COVID-19 pediatric patients who later develop severe MIS-C, Weisberg and colleagues[40] measured anti-S and anti-N IgG, IgA, and IgM antibody responses in 13 adults (median age 62) with COVID-19 and acute respiratory distress syndrome (COVID-ARDS) and 47 children (median age 11) with and without MIS-C. Although anti-S IgG, IgA, and IgM antibodies were elevated in adult patients with ARDS compared with patients without ARDS, all antibody classes showed similar levels for pediatric patients with and without MIS-C. Anti-N IgG responses were lower in pediatric patients compared with adult patients and were not dependent on disease severity in either adult or pediatric cohorts, suggesting that anti-N IgG production is age-dependent. In contrast, other studies have shown that antibody responses correlate with MIS-C severity. Pierce and colleagues[41] observed that patients with MIS-C had a larger ratio of IgG1 versus IgG3 compared with non-MIS-C patients. In a study with 192 enrolled pediatric participants, Yonker and colleagues[42] similarly reported that anti-RBD IgM and IgG antibodies were significantly increased in MIS-C patients compared with non-MIS-C patients. Children with acute COVID-19 and MIS-C had detectable IgM and IgG anti-RBD antibodies, as expected. Mild MIS-C pediatric patients showed low anti-RBD IgM and IgG levels. Notably, severe MIS-C cases showed elevated IgG levels against other coronaviruses

(229E, NL63, HKU1, and OC43), whereas mild MIS-C pediatric, COVID-19 adult, and recovered adult patients did not show such nonspecific antibody responses. These studies suggest that antibody subtype, antigen target, and humoral kinetics play a role in immunity in children. Future studies on significantly large cohorts are critical to further understand the relationship between humoral responses and COVID-19/MIS-C pathologic condition in children.

Humoral Immunity During Convalescence

Mounting evidence suggests that high antibody responses persist for several months after COVID-19 patients reach convalescence.[25,27,43–45] In a longitudinal cohort of 250 convalescent patients, Boonyaratanakornkit and colleagues[43] observed high anti-S1 IgG antibodies lasting several months ($t_{1/2} \sim$ 66.2 days) that correlated with neutralization titers. Similarly, a study of 43 COVID-19-positive patients showed 95% maintenance of anti-RBD IgG levels and neutralization titers at 6 months after symptom onset ($t_{1/2} \sim$ 140 days).[46] A large-scale study in 30,082 COVID-19 patients showed high anti-S1 IgG and neutralization titers lasting 5 months after infection.[44] However, studies have also shown that antibody levels decline after infection. In a longitudinal study of anti-N and anti-S IgG, anti-S1 and anti-RBD IgA, and anti-S1 and anti-RBD IgM levels in 26 health care workers, Marot and colleagues[45] observed waning of IgA antibodies 2 months after disease onset, whereas IgG and IgM levels persisted for 3 months. Decline of anti-S, anti-N, and anti-RBD IgG, IgA, and IgM were similarly observed 3 months after infection by Seow and colleagues,[47] which correlated with a decline in neutralizing antibody responses.

The risk of reinfection in convalescent COVID-19 individuals with or without maintenance of antibody titers remains a major unknown in the COVID-19 pandemic. Lumley and colleagues[48] measured anti-S and anti-N IgG antibodies across 12,541 health care workers in the United Kingdom over 7 months and defined reinfection as the first positive PCR test at least 60 days after an initial positive antibody test. Individuals who were initially seropositive for anti-S and anti-N IgG antibodies presented a substantially lower rate of reinfection than individuals who were initially seronegative. These results agree with work from Hall and colleagues,[49] who found that 30,625 health care workers with previous SARS-CoV-2 infection were at 84% lower risk of reinfection than workers without previous infection. Of note, Lee and colleagues[50] presented a case study of one patient who mounted robust anti-RBD and anti-S1 IgG responses to SARS-CoV-2 but, despite maintaining antibody seropositivity, was reinfected with SARS-CoV-2 26 days after initial infection. Evidence of SARS-CoV-2 reinfection in previously infected individuals indicates that antibody markers may not be sufficient to predict immunity to SARS-CoV-2. Although it is now possible to perform serologic studies in individuals over 1 year after SARS-CoV-2 infection, these studies are yet to be reported, and mechanisms of long-term humoral immunity remain unknown.

SUMMARY

Studies on humoral responses to SARS-CoV-2 have been reported with unprecedented speed and with resolution that enables analysis of specific antigen-antibody interactions during all stages of infection and recovery. The authors present a review of literature on antigen targets for antibody responses in the context of acute immunity, clinical relevance, and convalescent immunity. S, N, and RBD proteins have been identified as key antigens in IgG, IgA, and IgM antibody responses during COVID-19 infection. Analysis of antigen-antibody responses continues to be critical in understanding COVID-19, especially in the context of vaccine development and viral variants. As COVID-19 vaccines are distributed, the ability to detect antigen-specific antibodies will be key in identifying individuals who have seroconverted from natural infected versus vaccination. For example, messenger RNA vaccines encode for S protein, and therefore, detection of antibodies against N protein would signify seropositivity from natural SARS-CoV-2 infection. Another key question is whether individuals with SARS-CoV-2 antibodies, either by vaccination or by natural infection, will be immune from reinfection by SARS-CoV-2 variants. Mutations for several variants have been identified on the S protein, specifically the RBD region.[51] New assays for detection of antibodies against antigen variants will be key to further understanding humoral responses to SARS-CoV-2 as the virus evolves.

CLINICS CARE POINTS

- Point-of-care SARS-CoV-2 antibody testing is effective in identifying antibodies from previus infections in mildly and severely symptomatic individuals.
- Monitoring patient seroconversion can effectively guide clinicians to assess COVID-19 disease severity and implementent suitable therapeutics.
- Quantifying antibody levels via point-of-care serology tests as a screen for prior infection can enable clinicians to evaluate effective timepoints for administration of vaccines and boosters for healthy and immunocompromised individuals.
- Monitoring overall seroconversion in a population provides data for disease epidemiology and outbreak containment measures.

DISCLOSURE

D.R. Walt has a financial interest in Quanterix Corporation, a company that develops an ultrasensitive digital immunoassay platform. He is an inventor of the Simoa technology, founder of the company, and serves on its Board of Directors. Dr D.R. Walt's interests were reviewed and are managed by Brigham and Women's Hospital and Partners HealthCare in accordance with their conflict-of-interest policies.

REFERENCES

1. Burrell CJ, Howard CR, Murphy FA. Coronaviruses. Fenner White's Med Virol 2017;437–46. https://doi.org/10.1016/B978-0-12-375156-0.00031-X.
2. Hu B, Guo H, Zhou P, et al. Characteristics of SARS-CoV-2 and COVID-19. Nat Rev Microbiol 2021;19:141–54.
3.. Shang J, Wan Y, Luo C, et al. Cell entry mechanisms of SARS-CoV-2. Proc Natl Acad Sci U S A 2020;117.
4. Chilamakuri R, Agarwal S. COVID-19: characteristics and therapeutics. Cells 2021;10:1–29.
5. Neurath AR. Immune response to viruses: antibody-mediated immunity. Encycl Virol 2008;56–70.
6. GeurtsvanKessel CH, Okba NMA, Igloi Z, et al. An evaluation of COVID-19 serological assays informs future diagnostics and exposure assessment. Nat Commun 2020;11:1–5.
7. Schroeder HW Jr, Cavacini L. Structure and function of immunoglobulins. J Allergy Clin Immunol 2010;125:S41–52.

8. Casali P, Schettino EW. Structure and function of natural antibodies. In: Potter M, Rose NR, editors. Immunology of Silicones, 167–179. Springer Berlin Heidelberg; 1996.

9. Grönwall C, Vas J, Silverman G. Protective roles of natural IgM antibodies. Front Immunol 2012;3:66.

10. Skountzou I, Satyabhama L, Stavropoulou A, et al. Influenza virus-specific neutralizing IgM antibodies persist for a lifetime. Clin Vaccin Immunol. 2014;21: 1481–9.

11. Krammer F. The human antibody response to influenza A virus infection and vaccination. Nat Rev Immunol 2019;19:383–97.

12. Maurer MA, Meyer L, Bianchi M, et al. Glycosylation of human IgA directly inhibits influenza A and other sialic-acid-binding viruses. Cell Rep 2018;23:90–9.

13. Rikhtegaran Tehrani Z, Saadat S, Saleh E, et al. Performance of nucleocapsid and spike-based SARS-CoV-2 serologic assays. PLoS One 2020;15:e0237828.

14. Van Elslande J, Decru B, Jonckheere S, et al. Antibody response against SARS-CoV-2 spike protein and nucleoprotein evaluated by four automated immunoassays and three ELISAs. Clin Microbiol Infect 2020;26:1557.e1–7.

15. Long QX, Liu BZ, Wu GC, et al. Antibody responses to SARS-CoV-2 in patients with COVID-19. Nat Med 2020;26(6):845–8.

16. Guo L, Ren L, Yang S, et al. Profiling early humoral response to diagnose novel coronavirus disease (COVID-19). Clin Infect Dis Off Publ Infect Dis Soc Am 2020;71:778–85.

17. Grzelak L, Temmam S, Planchais C, et al. A comparison of four serological assays for detecting anti–SARS-CoV-2 antibodies in human serum samples from different populations. Sci Transl Med 2020;12(559):eabc3103.

18. Corthésy B. Role of secretory IgA in infection and maintenance of homeostasis. Autoimmun Rev 2013;6:661–5.

19. Long Q-X, Tang XJ, Shi QL, et al. Clinical and immunological assessment of asymptomatic SARS-CoV-2 infections. Nat Med 2020;26:1200–4.

20. Guthmiller JJ, Stovicek O, Wang J, et al. SARS-CoV-2 infection severity is linked to superior humoral immunity against the spike. MBio 2021;12:1–13.

21. Legros V, Denolly S, Vogrig M, et al. A longitudinal study of SARS-CoV-2-infected patients reveals a high correlation between neutralizing antibodies and COVID-19 severity. Cell. Mol. Immunol. 2021;18:318–27.

22. Atyeo C, Fischinger S, Zohar T, et al. Distinct early serological signatures track with SARS-CoV-2 survival. Immunity 2020;53:524–32.e4.

23. Rogers TF, Zhao F, Huang D, et al. Isolation of potent SARS-CoV-2 neutralizing antibodies and protection from disease in a small animal model. Science 2020; 369(6506):956–63.

24. Premkumar L, Segovia-Chumbez B, Jadi R, et al. The receptor-binding domain of the viral spike protein is an immunodominant and highly specific target of antibodies in SARS-CoV-2 patients. Sci Immunol 2020;5:1–10.

25. Cao Y, Su B, Guo X, et al. Potent neutralizing antibodies against SARS-CoV-2 identified by high-throughput single-cell sequencing of convalescent patients' B cells. Cell 2020;182:73–84.e16.

26. Rydyznski Moderbacher C, Ramirez S, Dan J, et al. Antigen-specific adaptive immunity to SARS-CoV-2 in acute COVID-19 and associations with age and disease severity. Cell 2020;183:996–1012.e19.

27. Garcia-Beltran WF, Lam E, Astudillo M, et al. COVID-19-neutralizing antibodies predict disease severity and survival. Cell 2021;184:476–88.e11.

28. Suhandynata RT, Hoffman M, Huang D, et al. Commercial serology assays predict neutralization activity against SARS-CoV-2. Clin Chem 2021;67:404–14.

29. Indenbaum V, Koren R, Katz-likvornik S, et al. Testing IgG antibodies against the RBD of SARS-CoV-2 is sufficient and necessary for COVID-19 diagnosis. PLoS One 2020;15:e0241164.

30. Mekonnen D, Mengist HM, Derbie A, et al. Diagnostic accuracy of serological tests and kinetics of severe acute respiratory syndrome coronavirus 2 antibody: a systematic review and meta-analysis. Rev Med Virol 2020;31(3):e2181.

31. Röltgen K, Powell AP, Wirz OF, et al. Defining the features and duration of antibody responses to SARS-CoV-2 infection associated with disease severity and outcome. Sci Immunol 2021;5:1–20.

32. Suthar MS, Zimmerman MG, Kauffman RC, et al. Rapid generation of neutralizing antibody responses in COVID-19 patients. Cell Rep Med 2020;1:100040.

33. Ravichandran S, Lee Y, Grubbs G, et al. Longitudinal antibody repertoire in "mild" versus "severe" COVID-19 patients reveals immune markers associated with disease severity and resolution. Sci Adv 2021;7:1–16.

34. Bartsch YC, Wang C, Zohar T, et al. Humoral signatures of protective and pathological SARS-CoV-2 infection in children. Nat Med 2021;27:454–62.

35. Li K, Huang B, Zhong A, et al. Dynamic changes in anti-SARS-CoV-2 antibodies during SARS-CoV-2 infection and recovery from COVID-19. Nat Commun 2020; 11:6044.

36. Markewitz R, Torge A, Wandinger KP, et al. Clinical correlates of anti-SARS-CoV-2 antibody profiles in Spanish COVID-19 patients from a high incidence region. Sci Rep 2021;11:4363.

37. Norman M, Gilboa T, Ogata AF, et al. Ultrasensitive high-resolution profiling of early seroconversion in patients with COVID-19. Nat Biomed Eng 2020;4:1180–7.

38. Ogata AF, Maley AM, Wu C, et al. Ultra-sensitive serial profiling of SARS-CoV-2 antigens and antibodies in plasma to understand disease progression in COVID-19 patients with severe disease. Clin Chem 2020. https://doi.org/10.1093/clinchem/hvaa213.

39. Lucas C, Klein J, Sundaram M, et al. Kinetics of antibody responses dictate COVID-19 outcome. medRxiv 2020.

40. Weisberg SP, et al. Distinct antibody responses to SARS-CoV-2 in children and adults across the COVID-19 clinical spectrum. Nat Immunol 2021;22:25–31.

41. Pierce CA, Preston-Hurlburt P, Dai Y, et al. Immune responses to SARS-CoV-2 infection in hospitalized pediatric and adult patients. Sci Transl Med 2020; 12(564):eabd5487.

42. Yonker LM, Neilan AM, Bartsch Y, et al. Pediatric severe acute respiratory syndrome coronavirus 2 (SARS-CoV-2): clinical presentation, infectivity, and immune responses. J Pediatr 2020;227:45–52.e5.

43. Boonyaratanakornkit J, Morishima C, Selke S, et al. Clinical, laboratory, and temporal predictors of neutralizing antibodies against SARS-CoV-2 among COVID-19 convalescent plasma donor candidates. J Clin Invest 2021;131(3):e144930.

44. Wajnberg A, Amanat F, Firpo A, et al. Robust neutralizing antibodies to SARS-CoV-2 infection persist for months. Science 2020;370:1227–30.

45. Marot S, Malet I, Leducq V, et al. Rapid decline of neutralizing antibodies against SARS-CoV-2 among infected healthcare workers. Nat Commun 2021;12:1–7.

46. Dan JM, Mateus J, Kato Y, et al. Immunological memory to SARS-CoV-2 assessed for up to 8 months after infection. Science 2021;80-:371.

47. Seow J, Graham C, Merrick B, et al. Longitudinal observation and decline of neutralizing antibody responses in the three months following SARS-CoV-2 infection in humans. Nat Microbiol 2020;5:1598–607.
48. Lumley SF, O'Donnell D, Stoesser N, et al. Antibody status and incidence of SARS-CoV-2 infection in health care workers. N Engl J Med 2021;384:533–40.
49. Hall VJ, Foulkes S, Charlett A, et al. SARS-CoV-2 infection rates of antibody-positive compared with antibody-negative health-care workers in England: a large, multicentre, prospective cohort study (SIREN). Lancet 2021;397:1459–69.
50. Lee JS, Kim SY, Hong KH, et al. Evidence of severe acute respiratory syndrome coronavirus 2 reinfection after recovery from mild coronavirus disease 2019. Clin Infect Dis 2020;1–7.
51. Wang R, Chen J, Gao K, et al. Analysis of SARS-CoV-2 mutations in the United States suggests presence of four substrains and novel variants. Commun Biol 2021;4:228.

Vaccine-Induced Severe Acute Respiratory Syndrome Coronavirus 2 Antibody Response and the Path to Accelerating Development (Determining a Correlate of Protection)

Amy C. Sherman, MD[a,b,1,*], Michaël Desjardins, MD[a,b,c,1], Lindsey R. Baden, MD[a,b]

KEYWORDS

- SARS-CoV-2 • Vaccines • Serologic diagnostics

KEY POINTS

- A marker of immunity that describes clinical efficacy for SARS-CoV-2 vaccines would be a valuable clinical and epidemiological tool.
- A "correlate" or "surrogate" of SARS-CoV-2 vaccine-induced protection needs to be well-defined, including clear endpoints (e.g., hospitalization, severe disease, transmission).
- Different statistical models and methodologies can be used to determine a correlate or surrogate of protection.
- Many factors including host characteristics, vaccine platform, and immunologic parameters may impact the correlate or surrogate of protection.

INTRODUCTION

Less than 18 months after the identification of severe acute respiratory syndrome coronavirus 2 (SARS-CoV-2) and its genome, 13 authorized or approved COVID-19 vaccines are being deployed around the world,[1] and many more candidates are currently undergoing evaluation in clinical trials. In the United States, 3 vaccines have been granted an Emergency Use Authorization (EUA) by the Food and Drug

[a] Division of Infectious Diseases, Brigham and Women's Hospital, 75 Francis Street, Boston, MA 02115, USA; [b] Harvard Medical School, Boston, MA 02115, USA; [c] Division of Infectious Diseases, Centre Hospitalier de l'Université de Montréal, 1000 Rue Saint-Denis, Bureau F06.1102b, Montreal, Quebec H2X 0C1, Canada
[1] Co-first authors.
* Corresponding author. Division of Infectious Diseases, Brigham and Women's Hospital, 75 Francis Street, Boston, MA 02115, USA
E-mail address: acsherman@bwh.harvard.edu

Clin Lab Med 42 (2022) 111–128
https://doi.org/10.1016/j.cll.2021.10.008
0272-2712/22/© 2021 Elsevier Inc. All rights reserved.
labmed.theclinics.com

Administration: BNT162b2 (Pfizer/BioNTech), mRNA-1273 (Moderna), and Ad26.CoV2.S (Janssen Biotech, Inc). Although the phase 3 clinical trials have demonstrated clinical efficacy in preventing moderate to severe COVID-19 disease, the underlying immune mechanisms that confer protection are still not known. Furthermore, determining protection against SARS-CoV-2 infection in vaccinated people using laboratory markers would be extremely useful. Efficacy studies, such as randomized controlled trials (RCTs), depend on large and expensive clinical trials, whereas large population studies during vaccine rollout often have confounding variables. Using a "surrogate" or "correlate" of protection allows for easier monitoring and surveillance of a particular vaccine's effectiveness, which can aid in both vaccine development and licensure.[2] Markers of immune responses can also be applied to determine a population response for new variants or strains of a virus, across unique characteristics of a population (eg, elderly, immunocompromised), and across different manufacturing or lots. Furthermore, COVID-19 vaccine boosters may be necessary, and a correlate of protection (CoP) would allow for efficient measurement of persistent protection. To date, there is no accepted CoP for COVID-19 vaccine-induced immunity.

The current knowledge regarding antibody-induced responses to SARS-CoV-2 vaccines, the definition of a CoP, proposed CoP for SARS-CoV-2, and special considerations for defining an SARS-CoV-2 vaccine-induced CoP are discussed.

SEVERE ACUTE RESPIRATORY SYNDROME CORONAVIRUS 2 VACCINES AND ANTIBODY RESPONSES

The varied COVID-19 vaccines that have been approved for emergency use or are still undergoing clinical evaluation use different technologies, administration schedules, and antigen targets (**Table 1**), which may result in different cellular and humoral responses following immunization. The available data on the dynamics, duration, and magnitude of the antibody responses following COVID-19 immunization are discussed in relation to different vaccine platforms.

Antibody responses to COVID-19 vaccines are commonly reported using 2 different assays: immunoassays to detect binding antibodies (bAb) and neutralization assays to detect neutralizing antibodies (nAb).[3] Immunoassays, such as enzyme-linked immunosorbent assays (ELISA), detect and quantify antibodies that have the capacity to bind a specific antigen in vitro. Except for inactivated vaccines, all available COVID-19 vaccines target the SARS-CoV-2 spike protein or one of its components (eg, receptor binding domain or RBD, S1, S2). Thus, it is expected that these vaccines will lead to the production of bAb against the spike protein, but not against the nucleocapsid protein. This antibody response signature is different from what is seen after natural infection or vaccination with inactivated vaccines, where detection of both spike and other antigens (such as nucleocapsid) bAb is expected. Neutralization assays are used to quantify functional antibodies that have the capacity to inhibit the replication of SARS-CoV-2 in vitro. Alternatively, a pseudovirus expressing SARS-CoV-2 spike protein can be used instead of wild-type SARS-CoV-2, providing significant safety and versatility advantages. In most phase 1/2 trials, a strong correlation was seen between bAb and nAb elicited postvaccination.[4–7]

Dynamics of Antibody Responses Postvaccination

In participants without previous SARS-CoV-2 infection, bAb, such as immunoglobulin G (IgG) against the full spike, S1, S2, or RBD, are usually detectable 14 days after the initial dose and tend to further increase on days 21 to 28, when the second dose is

Table 1
Vaccine platforms, dose and schedule, and antigen targets

Vaccine Platform	Vaccine Name	Approved/Authorized	Vaccine Dose and Schedule	Antigen Target
mRNA-based vaccines	BNT162b2 (Pfizer/BioNTech)	≥85 countries US EUA 12/11/2020	30 µg, 2 doses, 21 d apart[9]	Prefusion-stabilized full-length S protein
	mRNA-1273 (Moderna)	≥46 countries US EUA 12/18/2020	100 µg, 2 doses, 28 d apart[5,11,85]	Prefusion-stabilized full-length S protein
Vector vaccines	AZD1222 (Astra-Zeneca) Vector: ChAdeno	≥139 countries Not in the US	5×10^{10} VP, 2 doses, 4–12 wk apart[8,86]	Full-length S protein
	Ad26.CoV2.S (Janssen) Vector: Ad26	≥41 countries USA EUA 2/27/2021	5×10^{10} VP, 1 dose[4]	Prefusion-stabilized full-length S protein
	Sputnik V (Gamaleya Center) Vector: rAd26/rAd5	≥65 countries Not in the US	10^{11} VP, 2 doses 21 d apart[6]	Full-length S protein
	Convidicea (CanSino) Vector: rAd5	≥5 countries Not in the US	5×10^{10} VP, 1 dose[7]	Full-length S protein
Inactivated vaccines	CoronaVac (Sinovac)	≥24 countries Not in the US	3 µg, 2 doses 14–28 d apart[10,87]	Inactivated SARS-CoV-2 (CN02 strain)
	BBIBP-CorV (Sinopharm)	≥40 countries Not in the US	4 µg, 2 doses 21–28 d apart[63]	Inactivated SARS-CoV-2 (HB02 strain)
	Covaxin (Bharat Biotech)	≥9 countries Not in the US	6 µg, 2 doses 28 d apart[15,88]	Inactivated SARS-CoV-2 (NIV-2020-770 strain)
	WIBP-CorV (Sinopharm)	2 countries Not in the US	5 µg, 2 doses 21 d apart[89]	Inactivated SARS-CoV-2 (WIV04 strain)
	CoviVac (Chumakov Center)	1 country Not in the US	N/A, 2 doses, 14 d apart	Inactivated SARS-CoV-2 (strain N/A)
Subunit vaccine	EpiVacCorona (Vector Institute)	2 countries Not in the US	N/A, 2 doses 21–28 d apart (NCT04780035)	Synthesized peptide antigens of SARS-CoV-2
	ZF2001 (Anhui Zhifei Longcom Biopharmaceutical)	2 countries Not in the US	25 µg, 3 doses, 0–30–60 d[16]	Receptor-binding domain

administered.[5,8] All the 2-dose schedule vaccines show a *prime-boost* effect, with further significant increase of bAb peaking around 7 to 14 days after the second dose.[5,9,10]

In general, nAb are detected at a low level starting at day 14 and significantly increase after the second dose.[5,6,8] nAb tend to increase at a rate slower than bAb, however, like bAb, tend to peak 7 to 14 days postdosing schedule. The single-dose vaccines Ad26.CoV2.S (Janssen Biotech, Inc), a nonreplicating adenovirus serotype 26 (Ad26) vector vaccine, and Convidicea (CanSino), a nonreplicating adenovirus serotype 5 vector vaccine, produce bAb and nAb by day 28, that tend to further increase by day 56 for Ad26.CoV2.S.[4,7]

Limited data are available regarding the duration of antibody responses post-COVID-19 vaccines. Data generated from the phase 1 and phase 3 clinical trials are critical to better understand the duration of protection, as participants in these trials were vaccinated as early as March 2020 and July 2020, respectively. This prolonged follow-up period provides early understanding of the kinetics of antibody response and vaccine efficacy over time and may guide the need for future booster dose. In the mRNA-173 phase 1 study, in which 33 participants received 2 doses of vaccine 28 days apart, bAb and nAb titers decreased but persisted through 6 months after the second dose as assessed by 3 different assays.[11] There is also growing evidence from the phase 3 trials that vaccination with messenger RNA (mRNA) vaccines remains clinically effective to prevent confirmed symptomatic cases of COVID-19 for at least 6 months.[12,13]

Magnitude of Antibody Responses

The magnitude of postvaccination bAb and nAb published to date is difficult to compare between COVID-19 vaccine types, because researchers use different assays and methods to quantitate antibody levels. Furthermore, for bAb, assays target different antigens, such as the full spike protein or one of its fragments (S1, S2, RBD).[14] For this reason, some groups have included a panel of control convalescent serum specimen from individuals with prior COVID-19 to compare the vaccine-induced responses with the natural infection. mRNA and vector vaccines were shown to induce bAb and nAb titers similar to or higher than what is detected in convalescent sera.[4,5,8,9] For inactivated vaccines, only CoronaVac and Covaxin trials reported comparison with convalescent sera and showed respectively lower or similar nAb titers in sera from vaccinated participants compared with convalescents sera.[15] The recombinant vaccine ZF2001 showed significantly higher nAb titers in vaccinated participants than in convalescent sera.[16] However, these data must be cautiously interpreted because the serum panels differ among the different studies. Antibody titers after natural infection can vary significantly in convalescent individuals, based on host's characteristics, severity of disease, and timing from symptom onset.[3,17]

Impact of Previous Infection on Antibody Responses to Vaccines

In individuals with previous SARS-CoV-2 infection, postvaccination humoral responses differ significantly in terms of dynamics and magnitude. In those who received BNT162b2 (Pfizer, Inc) or mRNA-1273 (ModernaTx, Inc), a rapid increase of bAb is seen after the first dose, starting as early as 5 to 8 days.[18] The titers quickly peak at high levels between days 9 and 12 and do not significantly increase after the second dose. In comparison with those without preexisting immunity, the titers were 10 to 45 times higher after the first dose and remained 6 times higher after the second dose. Another study showed that 2 doses of BNT162b2 (Pfizer, Inc) in previously uninfected individuals induced lower nAb titers than a single dose in those with previous infection.

COVID-19 Vaccines Humoral Responses and Variants

In the early phase 1/2 COVID-19 vaccine trials, vaccine-induced neutralizing activity was assessed by neutralization assays using pseudovirus expressing the wild-type Spike protein or using wild-type SARS-CoV-2. However, since January 2021, many different genetic variants of SARS-CoV-2 have emerged around the world. These variants have various substitutions, insertions, and/or deletions in the spike protein gene that may lead to increased transmissibility or disease severity, and may also reduce vaccine-induced protection.[19] Current variants of concern according to the Centers for Disease Control and Prevention include B.1.1.7 (first identified in United Kingdom), P1 (first identified in Brazil), B1.351 (first identified in South Africa), and B.1.427 and B.1.429 (first identified in California, USA). Emerging data have shown reduced, but variable neutralizing activity of postvaccination sera on these variants, with a small to moderate reduction in activity on the B.1.1.7, P1, B.1.427, and B.1.429,[20,21] and more significant reduction of neutralization was shown on the B1.351 variant, particularly with AZD1222, where complete virus escape has been described.[22] In patients with previous SARS-CoV-2 infection, a single dose of BNT162b2 substantially increased the serum neutralizing activity against B.1.1.7, P1, and B.1.351, with similar titers across patients for each variant.[23]

DEFINITION AND HISTORICAL EXAMPLES OF CORRELATES OF PROTECTION AND RISKS

There are several definitions of the terms "correlate of protection" and "correlates of risk." Plotkin and Plotkin[24] define a CoP as "a specific immune response to a vaccine that is closely related to protection against infection, disease, or other defined end point." A CoP is typically a measurable immune marker, and preferably one that is relatively easy to obtain by standard laboratory techniques, for facile scalability and reproducibility. Importantly, Plotkin and Plotkin argue that the correlate itself confers protection, which they distinguish from a "surrogate," which is not itself protective but is an appropriate substitute for a different immune response that does offer protection. When defining a CoP, it is equally important to define the endpoint being described. For example, does the immunologic parameter provide protection against infection, transmission, hospitalization, or death? Depending on the outcome measure, the threshold value of a CoP may vary. The term "correlates of risk" was described by Qin and colleagues[25,26] as the statistical assessment of a CoP in the context of a clinical trial. In this assessment, the clinical endpoint is the outcome measure of efficacy as predetermined in the clinical trial.

The humoral immune response is an essential feature of protection for many vaccine-preventable diseases. Antibodies have been described as good correlates of protection for several different types of pathogens, including tetanus, pneumococcus, hepatitis A, hepatitis B, diphtheria, and *Haemophilus influenzae* b.[27–29] Passive immunity from transfer of antibodies can be shown to be protective. For example, antibodies transferred from maternal transmission to the fetus or antibodies provided clinically by injection can confer protection, which demonstrates a direct protective effect of the immune marker in question. Often, a discrete and quantitative antibody threshold value for protection can be described. However, it should be noted that antibody quality rather than quantity may also be important, and thus, a potential limitation in identifying a simplistic quantity of antibody as being protective for a given pathogen.

The immune system is complex and redundant. Thus, some have proposed that a CoP for a given vaccine is not reflective in a single immune marker, but rather could be a series of immune markers in an immune cascade, or numerous independent immune markers. For example, a clear correlate for measles protection has been identified, with an antibody level of plaque reduction neutralization greater than 120 mIU/mL, as demonstrated by successful protection with maternal-fetal transmission of antibodies.[30] However, individuals who are unable to produce antibodies because of humoral deficiencies can clear measles infection, demonstrating an alternative pathway of T-cell–induced immunity that confers protection.[31,32] Therefore, multiple immune pathways may be important for generating protection depending on the pathogen and characteristics of the host, with several unique correlates of protection.

Methods to Evaluate Immune Correlates

Much controversy exists in the literature regarding the meaning and utilization of immune-based correlates. A vaccine can be shown to induce a specific immune response; however, this does not necessarily translate to clinical efficacy. A vaccine may also have an immune response that is statistically associated with an assessment of efficacy; however, this value does not directly translate into a causal relationship between the immune marker and protection. To further refine how correlates should be described and thereby applied, several investigators have suggested validation models using a combination of statistical and clinical data.

Prentice[33] developed 4 criteria to evaluate endpoints for RCTs. These criteria have been adapted in the context of vaccine trials, as listed below[34]:

1. Protection against the clinical endpoint is significantly related to having received the vaccine.
2. The substitute endpoint is significantly related to the vaccination status.
3. The substitute endpoint is significantly related to protection against the clinical endpoint.
4. The full effect of the vaccine on the frequency of the clinical endpoint is explained by the substitute endpoint, as it lies on the sole causal pathway.

Although described specifically for RCTs, others have demonstrated that the Prentice criteria can also be applied for observational studies, although this was elucidated in relation to cancer research and not vaccinology research.[35]

Qin and colleagues[25] proposed a framework to statistically describe 3 different levels of correlates of protection and defined the data requirements needed to systematically validate the immune marker for each level. The 3 levels are defined as follows: (1) "correlate of risk," which is most closely associated with protection against a clinical outcome as determined in a clinical trial; followed by (2) "level 1 specific surrogate of protection" (further split between statistical and principal surrogates); and (3) "level 2 general surrogate of protection." Although "correlate of risk" was initially described in the context of a clinical trial, Qin's methods have been adapted for use in the setting of outbreak investigations, as with Ebola vaccinations in the Democratic Republic of the Congo.[36] Qin's "level 1" statistical category must adhere to the Prentice criteria, and "level 2" can be determined only through a large-scale phase 3 trial or large post-licensure studies that have the statistical power to calculate vaccine efficacy across populations.

The threshold method has also been described, in which a specific level of the immune marker is identified. Individuals who have values above the threshold are considered protected against the clinical endpoint, whereas those with levels below the threshold are susceptible.[29,37] Different statistical tests can estimate the threshold by either (1) comparing preexposure immune marker levels to disease incidence immune marker levels in observational/cohort studies or (2) examining the proportion of vaccinated and unvaccinated individuals below the threshold and calculating the immune marker-derived vaccine efficacy.[38,39] The threshold method and variations have been used to describe specific antibody-associated levels of protection for several vaccines, including the pneumococcal conjugate vaccine,[29] meningococcal C conjugate vaccine,[40] and rubella vaccine.[39]

Although the methodologies described by Prentice, Qin, and others can be valuable to statistically validate a CoP, the foundation rests on the measurement of the immunologic marker. Assays that have a wide degree of variability and measurement error will impact the subsequent statistical calculations used in these models. Measurement errors should be carefully considered for the SARS-CoV-2 antibody assays, which have shown varying degrees of sensitivity and specificity, with no gold standard, and with various types of assays used for different COVID-19 vaccine trials and post-EUA analyses.[41,42]

THE PATH TO DEFINING CORRELATE OF PROTECTION FOR SEVERE ACUTE RESPIRATORY SYNDROME CORONAVIRUS 2 VACCINES

Determining a CoP for SARS-CoV-2 is essential to determine both individual and population level immunity, and to describe protection both after natural infection and after vaccination. Furthermore, as new variants emerge and current vaccines are adapted, a defined CoP will be useful to efficiently generate and implement vaccination programs and identify novel vaccines for use in specific populations. As described above, an important factor in describing a CoP is defining and harmonizing the clinical or efficacy endpoint. A uniform endpoint for SARS-CoV-2 has not been clearly defined, with heterogeneous outcome measures described across clinical trials and other COVID-19 studies.[43] The current literature describes the insights gained from passive immunization of monoclonal antibodies in humans as well as possible correlates of protection as shown in animal models and cohort studies (summarized in **Table 2**). RCTs, large population observational studies, and challenge trials may also aid in identifying CoPs for SARS-CoV-2. Furthermore, as new SARS-CoV-2 variants emerge, sieve analyses may be used to better understand the mechanism behind vaccine protection by using genetic and statistical approaches to measure dissimilarity between virus strains in vaccinated individuals as compared with virus strains in placebo recipients.[44] Similar approaches have been used in the field of HIV-1 vaccines and prevention.[45]

Passive Immunity

described earlier, a true CoP is an immune component that is responsible for protection against a disease endpoint and can be demonstrated by passive transfer from an immune individual to a naïve individual. For SARS-CoV-2, monoclonal antibodies (mAb) have been developed that validate the role of neutralization antibodies as a mechanism of protection against disease.[46] A double-blind, phase 1 to 3 trial investigated the use of an antibody cocktail (REGN-COV2) in nonhospitalized, symptomatic patients.[47] The cocktail is composed of 2 neutralizing human IgG1 antibodies that target the RBD of SARS-CoV-2. The interim analysis demonstrated reduction of the SARS-CoV-2 viral load in participants who received the REGN-COV2 antibody cocktail, with a more pronounced effect in individuals who had not yet produced endogenous antibody. Another randomized, placebo-controlled phase 2 study (BLAZE-1) evaluated the role of LY-CoV555, an anti-spike neutralizing mAb that binds with high affinity to the RBD region of SARS-CoV-2 in patients with mild to moderate COVID-19 disease in the outpatient setting.[48] For one of the 3 dose levels tested, there

Table 2
Proposed correlates of protection

Study Design	Authors	Natural Infection or Postimmunization	Endpoint	Correlates of Protection Identified
Passive immunity	Weinreich et al,[47] 2021 Chen et al,[48] 2021	Passive antibody transfer	SARS-CoV-2 viral load	nAb, no specific threshold determined
Animal model	McMahan et al,[50] 2021	Natural infection	SARS-CoV-2 PCR detection in BAL	50 for pseudovirus nAb titers; 100 for RBD ELISA titers; 400 for S ELISA titers
Animal model	Corbett et al,[52] 2020	Postimmunization	SARS-CoV-2 PCR detection in BAL	nAb, no specific threshold determined
Animal model	Mercado et al,[51] 2020	Postimmunization	SARS-CoV-2 PCR detection in BAL	nAb 100–250
Cohort study	Addetia et al,[58] 2020	Natural infection	SARS-CoV-2 PCR (nasopharyngeal) and clinical symptoms	nAb were protective in 3 crew members with levels of 1:174, 1:161, and 1:3082

was a significant decline in viral load by day 11 as compared with the placebo group as well as a trend toward fewer hospitalizations and lower symptom burden in patients who received LY-CoV555. These data suggest a direct beneficial role of nAb in COVID-19. Studies are ongoing to better understand if mAb would also be beneficial in preventing SARS-CoV-2 infection in close contacts of infected individuals (eg, NCT04452318), which would provide additional insight into the role of humoral immunity in protection.

Animal Models

An animal model with rhesus macaques was developed and demonstrated SARS-CoV-2 infection and replication in pneumocytes and bronchial epithelial cells.[49] All macaques produced SARS-CoV-2 anti-spike bAb and nAb responses as well as SARS-CoV-2–specific cellular immune responses. After 35 days from the initial viral infection, the macaques were rechallenged with the same dose of SARS-CoV-2. Limited levels to no levels of viral RNA were detected from bronchoalveolar lavage (BAL) or nasal swabs in the rechallenged animals, which exhibited asymptomatic or mild clinical disease. These data suggest immunologic control upon rechallenge. However, because of the small sample size and near complete protection of the animals after rechallenge, no immune correlates of protection were identified. Given the positive responses of bAb, nAb, and cellular immune activation, the relative dominance of any one of these immune markers could not be determined.

The investigators next investigated the use of IgG transfer from convalescent macaque sera to naïve macaques who were subsequently challenged with SARS-CoV-2 as well as depletion of CD8+ T cells in convalescent macaques to identify a CoP.[50] The macaques who received the purified IgG were protected against the challenge infection in a dose-dependent manner. Using logistic regression models, antibody thresholds greater than 50 for pseudovirus nAb titers, 100 for RBD ELISA titers, and 400 for S ELISA titers were demonstrated to be protective. In the CD8+ T-cell–depleted group, some breakthrough infections occurred, suggesting that protection is not independently related to T-cell function, but that cellular immunity likely plays a role, especially in the setting of low antibody titers.

The same macaque model was then used to assess for vaccine-induced protection with DNA vaccine candidates and Ad26 vector vaccines.[51] Viral replication in BAL fluid and nasal secretions was measured for the endpoint analyses. Because of variability in the outcomes based on the different vaccine constructs administered, the investigators were able to evaluate for immune CoPs. An inverse correlation was described between nAb (both pseudovirus and live virus nAb titers) and RNA levels from BAL and nasal secretions, suggesting nAb as an immune CoP, with nAb titers between 100 and 250 offering complete protection.

Nonhuman primate challenge models have also been used to evaluate immune responses and determine CoP after vaccination. To evaluate CoP in the context of mRNA-1273 administration, nonhuman primates were challenged with intratracheal and intranasal SARS-CoV-2 four weeks after the second vaccination with mRNA-1273.[52] The endpoint assessment was quantification of SARS-CoV-2 RNA in BAL fluid and nasal secretions. mRNA-1273–induced serum neutralization activity was then correlated with RNA from BAL and nasal secretions and was found to be negatively correlated. Given this finding, in combination with the rapid reduction in viral replication 24 to 48 hours after challenge, the investigators speculated that antibodies do serve as the primary mechanism of protection. However, a specific threshold could not be determined, because the vaccine-induced immune response offered high protection with limited variation in viral replication.

A limitation of animal models is the inability to entirely recapitulate human pathogenesis and disease. The concentration and inoculation of virus for the challenge in animals may not reflect true transmission dynamics in humans.

Cohort and Observational Studies

Cohort and observational studies can provide information about CoP through epidemiologic analyses. Several cohort studies have examined rates of reinfection within distinct populations, which can also provide clues regarding CoP.[53–55] For example, a large, prospective cohort study in the United Kingdom, the SIREN (SARS-CoV-2 Immunity and Reinfection Evaluation) study, enrolled more than 30,000 health care workers and documented SARS-CoV-2 polymerase chain reaction (PCR) and antibody testing every 2 to 4 weeks.[56] The investigators describe that the seropositive participants (those with a prior history of SARS-CoV-2 infection) had an 84% lower risk of reinfection (adjusted incidence rate ratio 0.159; 95% CI 0.13–0.19). The data provide evidence that antibodies are protective against reinfection, although the investigators did not correlate specific antibody thresholds with protection.[57]

The outbreak that occurred on a fishery boat departing from Seattle was essential in determining that nAb were protective against SARS-CoV-2. One hundred three out of 117 individuals were seronegative before departure and were subsequently infected. Three members of the crew were seropositive with high nAb (1:174, 1:161, and 1:3082) before departure and did not develop infection as evidenced by negative SARS-CoV-2 PCR from nasopharyngeal swabs and lack of clinical symptoms.[58] Thus, high nAb were associated with protection, but no exact threshold could be determined from this observational study.

Challenge Studies

Human challenge studies involve the direct and controlled infection of healthy human volunteers and have been used to investigate novel vaccine candidates. Unlike RCTs or large population-based studies, controlled human challenge studies are faster and require fewer participants to measure efficacy and immune responses. These designs have been used to study other respiratory viral pathogens like influenza[59] and HCoV-229E and have been proposed to evaluate SARS-CoV-2.[60,61] Challenge models are attractive designs to determine immune CoP, because the exact timing of natural infection and/or immunization and dose can be tightly controlled, allowing for high-resolution assessment of correlations between immune markers and efficacy endpoints.

COVID-19 human challenge studies have begun in the United Kingdom.[62] The trials are currently ongoing; no data have been released yet regarding early findings. Later stages may offer insight to discerning CoP.

Randomized Controlled Trials

RCTs are well suited to define CoP, because clear clinical endpoints are established and measures of both vaccine efficacy and immune markers are documented at defined intervals. Using the threshold method and other statistical calculations, the vaccine efficacy can be correlated with an immune marker level to determine a CoP. Current evaluation of the phase 3 data is ongoing to determine a CoP, which may vary for different vaccine constructs.

OTHER CONSIDERATIONS RELATING TO CORRELATES OF PROTECTION

Based on correlates of protection for other infectious diseases, other important factors must be considered when defining immunologic markers of protection after COVID-19 vaccination. This section reviews some of these considerations, such as host factors, the vaccine platform and target antigen, and other important immunologic aspects of the immune response to vaccination.

Host Factors

Host factors, such as age, chronic medical conditions, and the use of immunosuppressive therapies, have been shown to impact the antibody responses to COVID-19 vaccines. These factors may also impact definitions of COVID-19 postvaccination correlates or surrogates of protection.

Age is an important factor influencing humoral vaccine responses. Most of the COVID-19 vaccine phase 1/2 trials showed that the magnitude of the vaccine-induced antibody responses in older individuals is generally lower than the antibody magnitude produced by younger individuals. For example, mRNA vaccines were shown to produce lower titers of bAb and lower or similar titers of nAb in participants older than 55 to 65 years of age.[5,9] The same tendency was shown with vector vaccines, except for AZD1222, which showed similar bAb and nAb titers in all age groups.[4,8,10] BBIP-CorV, an inactivated vaccine, led to lower nAb production in those aged 60 and older.[63]

The components of the immune response postvaccination that best correlate with protection may differ quantitively and qualitatively because of immunosenescence.[64] For example, in adults up to 50 years old, serum influenza hemagglutination inhibition levels of about 1:40 correlate well with protection.[24] However, higher postvaccination titers $\geq$1:40 are common among older individuals who develop influenza, suggesting that this threshold is not protective for older individuals.[65] In older individuals, T-cell responses may be a better correlate of vaccine protection against influenza.[66]

The effect of age on COVID-19 vaccine immune correlates is currently unknown. The correlation of bAb and nAb titers after Ad26.CoV2.S was stronger in younger individuals than in those 65 years and older.[4] This suggests a variation in the immune response phenotype in older individuals, which could influence the definition of immune correlates in this population.

Data are emerging regarding other host factors that are associated with lower humoral responses to COVID-19 vaccines, such as chronic comorbidities and immunocompromised states. For example, patients undergoing maintenance hemodialysis showed significant lower bAb than controls after 2 doses of BNT162b2.[67] Individuals with chronic inflammatory disease treated with immunosuppressive therapies, in particular those receiving B-cell depletion therapy of corticosteroids, exhibit significantly lower bAb and nAb titers after mRNA vaccines.[68] Solid organ transplant recipients were shown to have poor humoral responses after mRNA vaccines,[69,70] with older individuals and those receiving antimetabolite therapy having some of the poorest humoral responses.

Immunocompromised individuals have a significantly reduced humoral response to COVID-19 vaccines. CoP in this population may be different than in the general population. For example, patients treated with B-cell depletion therapy (anti-CD20) are usually unable to mount strong humoral immune responses to COVID-19 vaccines or SARS-CoV-2 infection.[71,72] However, infected individuals on such therapy still have the ability to clear the virus, which suggest that the cellular immune response or other arms of the immune system may have an important role.

Socioeconomic status, usually closely related to other factors, such as nutritional status, risk, and frequency of exposure, has been shown to impact immune correlates for other diseases. For example, the antibody titers associated with protection against pneumococcal infection has been shown to be higher among infants who live in low-resource settings.[29,73] The impact of socioeconomic status of environmental factors on correlates of protection from SARS-CoV-2 vaccination is unknown. However, because lower socioeconomic status has been already recognized as a risk factor for disease incidence and mortality,[74,75] it may be an important factor to consider as well when defining immune correlates after vaccination.

Vaccine Platform and Vaccine Antigens

Vaccines using different technological platforms and antigen targets may induce different qualitative and quantitative antibodies, which is another important factor to consider when establishing immune correlates for COVID-19 vaccines. This concept has been well described with other vaccines, such as those against *H influenzae* type b (polysaccharide vs conjugated vaccine) and *Bordetella pertussis* (whole cell vs acellular vaccine),[76,77] where different platforms were shown to yield different immune repertoire. COVID-19 vaccines use different technologies (mRNA, vector, subunit, inactivated) and different antigen targets (full spike, prefusion stabilized spike protein, RBD, inactivated virus), which may lead to different immune response quality and repertoire. Inactivated vaccines have the unique characteristic of presenting the whole virus to the immune system, which leads to the production of antibodies other than anti-spike, such as antinucleocapsid.[15] Even if the main target of nAb against SARS-CoV-2 appears to be the spike protein,[78] the antibody repertoire and diversity produced by inactivated vaccines may have immunologic significance against SARS-CoV-2 and the circulating variants that possess critical spike protein mutations.[79,80]

Immunologic Factors

The immune mechanisms leading to protection are complex and usually involve a combination of both humoral and cellular responses.[81] The impact of the relative importance of these 2 branches of the adaptive immune system for protection against SARS-CoV-2 is still unknown. Many studies have shown that antibodies are associated with protection against reinfection,[56] but few have evaluated the implication of cellular immune response on reinfection. COVID-19 vaccines have been shown to induce strong humoral immunity, but T-cell responses were also elicited after vaccination.[4,5] In a nonhumate primate study using an adenovirus-based vaccine (Ad26-S.PP), T-cell responses did not seem to correlate with protection.[51] It is still unknown if the cellular response contributes to protection in humans; however, there are clues that cellular responses are important. For example, the clinical protection from BNT162 against COVID-19 may start as soon as 12 days after the first dose.[82] However, nAb titers within the first 21 days after vaccination are low or undetectable.[9] Researchers showed that 3 weeks after the first BNT162b2 dose, nAb were not detected, but strong responses of RBD and spike antibodies with Fc-mediated effector functions and cellular responses largely by CD4[+] T-cell responses were seen.[83]

Mucosal immunity is another possible key component of COVID-19 protection, as SARS-CoV-2 initially infects the respiratory mucosal surfaces.[84] However, the mucosal immunity that results from COVID-19 natural infection and vaccination and its implication in defining COVID-19 correlates of protection remain largely unknown.

SUMMARY

The vaccine-induced CoP for SARS-CoV-2 has yet to be defined. When establishing a CoP, it will be essential not only to identify the appropriate immune marker but also to properly define the endpoint measure (eg, clinical disease, especially severe illness; transmission, SARS-CoV-2 PCR positivity) and understand the nuances of CoP in terms of host and antigen characteristics. Furthermore, standardized assays for the chosen immune marker or markers must be established in order to ensure comparability between disparate vaccine platforms and conditions of use. Ideally, these assays should be a test that is relatively easy to perform and does not require specialized equipment or reagents to promote easy scalability across the globe. Much of the focus has been to determine a humoral CoP, in part because of the ease of collection and evaluation, although cellular responses are also likely to be important.

As new public health challenges relating to COVID-19 emerge, such as variant strains, waning vaccine efficacy over time, and decreased vaccine efficacy for special populations (such as immunocompromised hosts), it is important to determine a CoP to allow accurate bridging studies for special populations and against variants of concern. In the context of a global pandemic with dynamic threats to public health, large-scale phase 3 clinical trials are inefficient to rapidly assess novel vaccine candidates for variant strains or for special populations, because these trials are slow and costly. Defining a practical CoP will aid in efficiently conducting future assessments to further describe protection for individuals and on a population level for surveillance.

CLINICS CARE POINTS

- The clinical utility of a correlate or surrogate of vaccine-induced immunity would be useful to assess individual and population-level protection, and allow for new vaccine candidates to be tested without costly and large efficacy trials.
- Further standardization of laboratory SARS-CoV-2 serologic tests are an equally important step to be able to use a correlate of protection in clinical practice.
- Clinicians and laboratorians must acknowledge that different vaccine platforms, circulating variants, and host factors may impact the correlate of the protection, and that a single marker of immunity may not be able specifically predict protection for all scenarios.

REFERENCES

1. COVID-19 vaccine tracker. Available at: https://www.raps.org/news-and-articles/news-articles/2020/3/covid-19-vaccine-tracker. Accessed April 25, 2021.
2. Plotkin SA. Immunologic correlates of protection induced by vaccination. Pediatr Infect Dis J 2001;20:63–75.
3. Immunogenicity of clinically relevant SARS-CoV-2 vaccines in nonhuman primates and humans | Science Advances. Available at: https://advances.sciencemag.org/content/7/12/eabe8065. Accessed April 25, 2021.
4. Sadoff J, Le Gars M, Shukarev G, et al. Interim results of a phase 1–2a trial of Ad26.COV2.S Covid-19 vaccine. New Engl J Med 2021;0. https://doi.org/10.1056/NEJMoa2034201.
5. Jackson LA, Anderson EJ, Rouphael NG, et al. An mRNA vaccine against SARS-CoV-2 — preliminary report. New Engl J Med 2020;0. https://doi.org/10.1056/NEJMoa2022483.
6. Logunov DY, Dolzhikova IV, Zubkova OV, et al. Safety and immunogenicity of an rAd26 and rAd5 vector-based heterologous prime-boost COVID-19 vaccine in two formulations: two open, non-randomised phase 1/2 studies from Russia. Lancet 2020;396:887–97.
7. Zhu F-C, Guan X-H, Li Y-H, et al. Immunogenicity and safety of a recombinant adenovirus type-5-vectored COVID-19 vaccine in healthy adults aged 18 years

or older: a randomised, double-blind, placebo-controlled, phase 2 trial. Lancet 2020;396:479–88.

8. Folegatti PM, Ewer KJ, Aley PK. Safety and immunogenicity of the ChAdOx1 nCoV-19 vaccine against SARS-CoV-2: a preliminary report of a phase 1/2, single-blind, randomised controlled trial. Lancet 2020;396:467–78.

9. Walsh EE, Frenck RW, Falsey AR, et al. Safety and immunogenicity of two RNA-based Covid-19 vaccine candidates. New Engl J Med 2020;383:2439–50.

10. Zhang Y, Zeng G, Pan H, et al. Safety, tolerability, and immunogenicity of an in-activated SARS-CoV-2 vaccine in healthy adults aged 18–59 years: a rando-mised, double-blind, placebo-controlled, phase 1/2 clinical trial. Lancet Infect Dis 2021;21:181–92.

11. Doria-Rose N, Suthar MS, Makowski M, et al. Antibody persistence through 6 months after the second dose of mRNA-1273 vaccine for Covid-19. New En-gland Journal of Medicine 2021. https://doi.org/10.1056/NEJMc2103916.

12. Pfizer and BioNTech confirm high efficacy and no serious safety concerns through up to six months following second dose in updated topline analysis of landmark COVID-19 vaccine study. 2021. Available at: https://www.businesswire.com/news/home/20210401005365/en/Pfizer-and-BioNTech-Confirm-High-Efficacy-and-No-Serious-Safety-Concerns-Through-Up-to-Six-Months-Following-Second-Dose-in-Updated-Topline-Analysis-of-Landmark-COVID-19-Vaccine-Study. Accessed May 3, 2021.

13. Moderna provides clinical and supply updates on COVID-19 vaccine program ahead of 2nd annual vaccines day | Moderna, Inc., (n.d.). Available at: https://investors.modernatx.com/news-releases/news-release-details/moderna-provides-clinical-and-supply-updates-covid-19-vaccine/. Accessed May 20, 2021.

14. Klasse PJ, Nixon DF, Moore JP. Immunogenicity of clinically relevant SARS-CoV-2 vaccines in nonhuman primates and humans. Sci Adv 2021;7:eabe8065.

15. Ella R, Reddy S, Jogdand H, et al. Safety and immunogenicity of an inactivated SARS-CoV-2 vaccine, BBV152: interim results from a double-blind, randomised, multicentre, phase 2 trial, and 3-month follow-up of a double-blind, randomised phase 1 trial. Lancet Infect Dis 2021. https://doi.org/10.1016/S1473-3099(21)00070-0.

16. Yang S, Li Y, Dai L, et al. Safety and immunogenicity of a recombinant tandem-repeat dimeric RBD-based protein subunit vaccine (ZF2001) against COVID-19 in adults: two randomised, double-blind, placebo-controlled, phase 1 and 2 trials. Lancet Infect Dis 2021. https://doi.org/10.1016/S1473-3099(21)00127-4.

17. Seow J, Graham C, Merrick B, et al. Longitudinal observation and decline of neutralizing antibody responses in the three months following SARS-CoV-2 infec-tion in humans. Nat Microbiol 2020;5:1598–607.

18. Krammer F, Srivastava K, Alshammary H, et al. Antibody responses in seroposi-tive persons after a single dose of SARS-CoV-2 mRNA vaccine. New Engl J Med 2021;384:1372–4.

19. CDC. Cases, Data, and surveillance. Centers for Disease Control and Prevention; 2020. Available at: https://www.cdc.gov/coronavirus/2019-ncov/cases-updates/variant-surveillance/variant-info.html. Accessed April 30, 2021.

20. Shen X, Tang H, Pajon R, et al. Neutralization of SARS-CoV-2 variants B.1.429 and B.1.351. New Engl J Med 2021;0. https://doi.org/10.1056/NEJMc2103740.

21. Wu K, Werner AP, Koch M, et al. Serum neutralizing activity elicited by mRNA-1273 vaccine. New Engl J Med 2021;384:1468–70.

22. Madhi SA, Baillie V, Cutland CL, et al. Efficacy of the ChAdOx1 nCoV-19 Covid-19 vaccine against the B.1.351 variant. New Engl J Med 2021;0. https://doi.org/10.1056/NEJMoa2102214.

23. Lustig Y, Nemet I, Kliker L, et al. Neutralizing response against variants after SARS-CoV-2 infection and one dose of BNT162b2. New Engl J Med 2021;0. https://doi.org/10.1056/NEJMc2104036.

24. Plotkin SA, Plotkin SA. Correlates of vaccine-induced immunity. Clin Infect Dis 2008;47:401–9. https://doi.org/10.1086/589862.

25. Qin L, Gilbert PB, Corey L, et al. A framework for assessing immunological correlates of protection in vaccine trials. J Infect Dis 2007;196:1304–12.

26. Plotkin SA, Gilbert PB. Nomenclature for immune correlates of protection after vaccination. Clin Infect Dis 2012;54:1615–7.

27. Denoël PA, Goldblatt D, de Vleeschauwer I, et al. Quality of the Haemophilus influenzae type b (Hib) antibody response induced by diphtheria-tetanus-acellular pertussis/Hib combination vaccines. Clin Vaccin Immunol 2007;14:1362–9.

28. Jack AD, Hall AJ, Maine N, et al. What level of hepatitis B antibody is protective? J Infect Dis 1999;179:489–92.

29. Siber GR, Chang I, Baker S, et al. Estimating the protective concentration of antipneumococcal capsular polysaccharide antibodies. Vaccine 2007;25:3816–26.

30. Chen RT, Markowitz LE, Albrecht P, et al. Measles antibody: reevaluation of protective titers. J Infect Dis 1990;162:1036–42.

31. Plebani A, Fischer MB, Meini A, et al. T cell activity and cytokine production in X-linked agammaglobulinemia: implications for vaccination strategies. Int Arch Allergy Immunol 1997;114:90–3.

32. Gans HA. Deficiency of the humoral immune response to measles vaccine in infants immunized at age 6 Months. JAMA 1998;280:527.

33. Prentice RL. Surrogate endpoints in clinical trials: definition and operational criteria. Stat Med 1989;8:431–40.

34. World Health Organization. Correlates of vaccine-induced protection: methods and implications. 2013. Available at: https://apps.who.int/iris/bitstream/handle/10665/84288/WHO_IVB_13.01_eng.pdf. Accessed April 13, 2021.

35. Schatzkin A, Freedman LS, Dorgan J, et al. Using and interpreting surrogate endpoints in cancer research. IARC Sci Publ.; 1997. p. 265–71.

36. Halloran ME, Longini IM, Gilbert PB. Designing a study of correlates of risk for Ebola vaccination. Am J Epidemiol 2020;189:747–54.

37. Chen X, Bailleux F, Desai K, et al. A threshold method for immunological correlates of protection. BMC Med Res Methodol 2013;13:29.

38. Siber GR. Methods for estimating serological correlates of protection. Dev Biol Stand 1997;89:283–96.

39. Skendzel LP. Rubella immunity. Defining the level of protective antibody. Am J Clin Pathol 1996;106:170–4.

40. Validation of serological correlate of protection for meningococcal C conjugate vaccine by using efficacy estimates from postlicensure surveillance in England, (n.d.). Available at: https://www.ncbi.nlm.nih.gov/pmc/articles/PMC193909/. Accessed April 15, 2021.

41. Galipeau Y, Greig M, Liu G, et al. Humoral responses and serological assays in SARS-CoV-2 infections. Front Immunol 2020;11. https://doi.org/10.3389/fimmu.2020.610688.

42. Whitman JD, Hiatt J, Mowery CT, et al. Evaluation of SARS-CoV-2 serology assays reveals a range of test performance. Nat Biotechnol 2020;38:1174–83.

43. Mehrotra DV, Janes HE, Fleming TR, et al. Clinical endpoints for evaluating efficacy in COVID-19 vaccine trials. Ann Intern Med 2020;174:221–8.
44. Rolland M, Gilbert PB. Sieve analysis to understand how SARS-CoV-2 diversity can impact vaccine protection. PLOS Pathog 2021;17:e1009406.
45. Corey L, Gilbert PB, Juraska M, et al. Two randomized trials of neutralizing antibodies to prevent HIV-1 acquisition. New Engl J Med 2021;384:1003–14.
46. Taylor PC, Adams AC, Hufford MM, et al. Neutralizing monoclonal antibodies for treatment of COVID-19. Nat Rev Immunol 2021;1–12.
47. Weinreich DM, Sivapalasingam S, Norton T, et al. REGN-COV2, a neutralizing antibody cocktail, in outpatients with Covid-19. New Engl J Med 2021;384:238–51.
48. Chen P, Nirula A, Heller B, et al. SARS-CoV-2 neutralizing antibody LY-CoV555 in outpatients with Covid-19. New Engl J Med 2021;384:229–37.
49. Chandrashekar A, Liu J, Martinot AJ, et al. SARS-CoV-2 infection protects against rechallenge in rhesus macaques. Science 2020;369:812–7.
50. McMahan K, Yu J, Mercado NB, et al. Correlates of protection against SARS-CoV-2 in rhesus macaques. Nature 2021;590:630–4.
51. Mercado NB, Zahn R, Wegmann F, et al. Single-shot Ad26 vaccine protects against SARS-CoV-2 in rhesus macaques. Nature 2020;586:583–8.
52. Corbett KS, Flynn B, Foulds KE, et al. Evaluation of the mRNA-1273 vaccine against SARS-CoV-2 in nonhuman primates. New Engl J Med 2020;383:1544–55.
53. Lumley SF, O'Donnell D, Stoesser NE, et al. Antibody status and incidence of SARS-CoV-2 infection in health care workers. New Engl J Med 2021;384:533–40.
54. Hansen CH, Michlmayr D, Gubbels SM, et al. Assessment of protection against reinfection with SARS-CoV-2 among 4 million PCR-tested individuals in Denmark in 2020: a population-level observational study. The Lancet 2021;397:1204–12.
55. Harvey RA, Rassen JA, Kabelac CA, et al. Association of SARS-CoV-2 seropositive antibody test with risk of future infection. JAMA Intern Med 2021. https://doi.org/10.1001/jamainternmed.2021.0366.
56. Hall VJ, Foulkes S, Charlett A, et al. SARS-CoV-2 infection rates of antibody-positive compared with antibody-negative health-care workers in England: a large, multicentre, prospective cohort study (SIREN). Lancet 2021;397:1459–69.
57. Krammer F. Correlates of protection from SARS-CoV-2 infection. Lancet 2021;397:1421–3.
58. Addetia A, Crawford KHD, Dingens A, et al. Neutralizing antibodies correlate with protection from SARS-CoV-2 in humans during a fishery vessel outbreak with a high attack rate. J Clin Microbiol 2020;58. https://doi.org/10.1128/JCM.02107-20.
59. Sherman AC, Mehta A, Dickert NW, et al. The future of flu: a review of the human challenge model and systems biology for advancement of influenza vaccinology. Front Cell. Infect. Microbiol. 2019;9. https://doi.org/10.3389/fcimb.2019.00107. Available at:.
60. Deming ME, Michael NL, Robb M, et al. Accelerating development of SARS-CoV-2 vaccines — the role for controlled human infection models. New Engl J Med 2020;383:e63.
61. Callow KA, Parry HF, Sergeant M, et al. The time course of the immune response to experimental coronavirus infection of man. Epidemiol Infect 1990;105:435–46.
62. Kirby T. COVID-19 human challenge studies in the UK. Lancet Respir Med 2020;8:e96.
63. Xia S, Zhang Y, Wang Y, et al. Safety and immunogenicity of an inactivated SARS-CoV-2 vaccine, BBIBP-CorV: a randomised, double-blind, placebo-controlled, phase 1/2 trial. The Lancet Infect Dis 2021;21:39–51.

64. Grubeck-Loebenstein B, Della Bella S, Iorio AM, et al. Immunosenescence and vaccine failure in the elderly. Aging Clin Exp Res 2009;21:201–9.

65. Gravenstein S, Drinka P, Duthie EH, et al. Efficacy of an influenza hemagglutinin-diphtheria toxoid conjugate vaccine in elderly nursing home subjects during an influenza outbreak. J Am Geriatr Soc 1994;42:245–51.

66. McElhaney JE, Xie D, Hager WD, et al. T cell responses are better correlates of vaccine protection in the elderly. J Immunol 2006;176:6333–9.

67. Grupper A, Sharon N, Finn T, et al. Humoral response to the Pfizer BNT162b2 vaccine in patients undergoing maintenance hemodialysis,. CJASN 2021. https://doi.org/10.2215/CJN.03500321.

68. Glucocorticoids and B Cell depleting agents substantially impair immunogenicity of mRNA vaccines to SARS-CoV-2 | medRxiv. Available at: https://www.medrxiv.org/content/10.1101/2021.04.05.21254656v2. Accessed April 30, 2021.

69. A. Grupper, L. Rabinowich, D. Schwartz, et al, Reduced humoral response to mRNA SARS-Cov-2 BNT162b2 vaccine in kidney transplant recipients without prior exposure to the virus, Am J Transplant. Available at: 10.1111/ajt.16615.

70. Boyarsky BJ, Werbel WA, Avery RK, et al. Immunogenicity of a single dose of SARS-CoV-2 messenger RNA vaccine in solid organ transplant recipients. JAMA 2021. https://doi.org/10.1001/jama.2021.4385.

71. Fallet B, Kyburz D, Walker UA. Mild course of COVID-19 and spontaneous virus clearance in a patient with depleted peripheral blood b cells due to rituximab treatment. Arthritis Rheumatol 2020;72:1581–2.

72. Herishanu Y, Avivi I, Aharon A, et al. Efficacy of the BNT162b2 mRNA COVID-19 vaccine in patients with chronic lymphocytic leukemia. Blood 2021. https://doi.org/10.1182/blood.2021011568.

73. Jódar L, Butler J, Carlone G, et al. Serological criteria for evaluation and licensure of new pneumococcal conjugate vaccine formulations for use in infants. Vaccine 2003;21:3265–72.

74. Karmakar M, Lantz PM, Tipirneni R. Association of social and demographic factors with COVID-19 incidence and death rates in the US. JAMA Netw Open 2021; 4:e2036462.

75. Clouston SAP, Natale G, Link BG. Socioeconomic inequalities in the spread of coronavirus-19 in the United States: a examination of the emergence of social inequalities. Soc Sci Med 2021;268:113554.

76. Edwards KM, Meade BD, Decker MD, et al. Comparison of 13 acellular pertussis vaccines: overview and serologic response. Pediatrics 1995;96:548–57.

77. Jelonek MT, Chang SJ, Chiu CY, et al. Comparison of naturally acquired and vaccine-induced antibodies to Haemophilus influenzae type b capsular polysaccharide. Infect Immun 1993;61:5345–50.

78. Barnes CO, Jette CA, Abernathy ME, et al. SARS-CoV-2 neutralizing antibody structures inform therapeutic strategies. Nature 2020;588:682–7.

79. Huang B, Dai L, Wang H, et al. Serum sample neutralisation of BBIBP-CorV and ZF2001 vaccines to SARS-CoV-2 501Y.V2. Lancet Microbe 2021;0. https://doi.org/10.1016/S2666-5247(21)00082-3.

80. Abdool Karim SS, de Oliveira T. New SARS-CoV-2 variants — clinical, public health, and vaccine implications. New Engl J Med 2021;0. https://doi.org/10.1056/NEJMc2100362.

81. Amanna IJ, Slifka MK. Contributions of humoral and cellular immunity to vaccine-induced protection in humans. Virology 2011;411:206–15.

82. Polack FP, Thomas SJ, Kitchin N, et al. Safety and efficacy of the BNT162b2 mRNA Covid-19 vaccine. New Engl J Med 2020;383:2603–15.

Printed and bound by CPI Group (UK) Ltd, Croydon, CR0 4YY

03/10/2024

01040404-0013